PELVIC INFLAMMATORY
DISEASE

OBSTETRICS AND GYNECOLOGY ADVANCES

Additional books and e-books in this series can be found on Nova's website under the Series tab.

OBSTETRICS AND GYNECOLOGY ADVANCES

PELVIC INFLAMMATORY DISEASE

DANIEL ABEHSERA
EDITOR

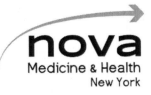

nova
Medicine & Health
New York

Copyright © 2019 by Nova Science Publishers, Inc.

Library of Congress Cataloging-in-Publication Data

ISBN: 978-1-53615-193-0

Published by Nova Science Publishers, Inc. † *New York*

CONTENTS

Preface   vii

Acronyms   xi

Chapter 1   Concept and Epidemiology   1
                Daniel Abehsera and Andrés C. López

Chapter 2   Clinical Manifestations and Diagnostic Criteria   11
                Laura Baños and Jessica Martín

Chapter 3   Microbiology of the Pelvic Inflammatory
                Disease: Molecular Biology Techniques   25
                Laura López and Paula Chamocho

Chapter 4   Risk Factors: Routes of Disease Transmission   39
                Marta de la Peña, Marta Casaus
                and Araceli Sánchez

Chapter 5   Complementary Tests in Pelvic
                Inflammatory Disease   55
                Raquel P. Duarte, Aurelia Marsac
                and Lourdes Martínez

Chapter 6   Pharmacological Treatment   **73**
                 Azucena Molina, Isabel Lozano
                 and Gemma Marín

Chapter 7   Surgical Treatment: The Role of Laparoscopy   **89**
                 Sadia Chocrón and Milagros Gálvez

Chapter 8   Complications and Consequences of Pelvic
                 Inflammatory Disease   **99**
                 Marta García and Celia Cuenca

Editor's Contact Information   **115**

Index   **117**

Related Nova Publications   **123**

PREFACE

Pelvic inflammatory disease (PID) is a disease that can occur in virtually all stages of woman's life. In addition, its variability in the expression of symptoms makes that the diagnosis is complex in many cases, leading to a delay in the treatment, with the consequent increase in the likelihood of sequelae. The objective of this monograph is to gather all the information available for the correct clinical management of all those situations in which an PID is presented. Eight chapters have been developed that address all aspects of PID, from basic notions to the most complicated aspects, in the diagnosis and treatment of PID.

Chapter 1: it is essential to have an exact knowledge of what PID is, since only in this way you can reach a correct diagnosis and treatment. It is necessary to know the structures of the female genital tract that may be involved, as well as the way in which the PID will affect them. It is also very important to know the epidemiology of the disease, since this will help us to differentiate the group of patients at risk, in which a PID can occur.

Chapter 2: the clinical manifestations of PID can alternate from a patient with a few symptoms to patients with a very suggestive exploration of a severe infectious disease. The need for diagnostic criteria is required, since in a high number of cases, the symptoms may not clearly reveal the presence of a PID. In fact, the presence of a diagnostic protocol is very important, to avoid that initial PID that go unnoticed, with the consequent increase in the morbidity of the disease.

Chapter 3: commonly the etiology of PID has been attributed to *Neisseria gonorrhoeae* and *Chlamydia trachomatis*. However, in a very large number of cases it is not possible to carry out an etiological diagnosis of the disease. This is mainly due to 2 reasons: on the one hand, a high number of cases of PID is caused by germs that are difficult to cultivate, such as *Mycoplasmas genitalium*; and on the other hand, the microbiological diagnosis of *Neisseria gonorrhoeae* and *Chlamydia trachomatis* is not simple. In addition, it is important to know the geographical distribution of this disease, since its incidence varies greatly in different countries.

Chapter 4: PID should be considered a sexually transmitted disease. In a large part of the cases, we find cases of PID in patients with other concomitant sexually transmitted diseases, and its incidence is directly related to the number of sexual partners that the patient presents. In addition, any pelvic surgery and / or instrumentation, such as the placement of an intrauterine device, is a predisposing factor to suffer a PID.

Chapter 5: the fact that in many cases of PID the disease is unclear, it is necessary in most clinical situations to perform complementary tests. In fact, the taking of samples for culture in order to look for the etiological agent, as well as the performance of a blood test to check the severity of the disease, is a must. In addition, on multiple occasions it is very useful to perform a CT scan of the abdomen and pelvis, because the symptoms presented by the patient are inconclusive. Magnetic resonance is also useful in cases in which there are doubts in the gynaecological ultrasound.

Chapter 6: the basis of the treatment of PID is the antibiotics. There are multiple proposed antibiotic regimens, which generally aim to reach all the germs that can produce a PID. The use of antibiotics empirically is due to the fact that the etiological diagnosis is usually delayed, and in many cases it is not possible to get to know which germ or germs have been responsible of the disease. Nor should we forget that PID always presents with pain, so a correct analgesic treatment is essential for a good management of the disease.

Chapter 7: When antibiotics fail or when the patient presents with pelvic peritonitis, surgical treatment is necessary for drainage and excision of possible pelvic abscesses. It is usually a difficult surgery, where anatomical planes are not well defined and multiple adhesions are generated. Laparoscopy is the route of choice, since in most cases it allows a complete treatment of the disease, although it is true that it requires well-trained surgeons in laparoscopic surgery.

Chapter 8: the PID can lead to very serious sequelae, which significantly compromise the patient's reproductive future, as well as their quality of life. In most cases there is an involvement of the fallopian tubes, and this fact implies that sterility of tubal origin is one of the main sequelae of PID; as well as tubal dysfunction leading to ectopic pregnancy. In addition, chronic pelvic pain can be a sequel of a PID, being a trouble of very difficult management and resolution.

ACRONYMS

AMR	Antimicrobial resistance
ART	Assisted reproductive technologies
CDC	Center for Disease Control and Prevention
CE	Chronic endometritis
CPP	Chronic pelvic pain
CRP	C-reactive protein
CT	Computerized tomography
ESR	Erythrocyte sedimentation rate
HMO	Health Maintenance Organization
HIV	Human immunodeficiency virus
IM	Intramuscular
IUD	Intrauterine device
IUSTI	International Union against Sexually Transmitted Infections
IV	Intravenous
IVF	In vitro fertilization
NAAT	Nucleic acid amplification test
OC	Oral contraceptives
PID	Pelvic inflammatory disease
PCR	Polymerase chain reaction
SDA	Strand displacement amplification

SPP	Species
STI	Sexually transmitted infection
TMA	Transcription - mediated amplification
TOA	Tubo – ovarian abscess
UK	United Kingdom
WHO	World Health Organization

In: Pelvic Inflammatory Disease   ISBN: 978-1-53615-193-0
Editor: Daniel Abehsera   © 2019 Nova Science Publishers, Inc.

Chapter 1

CONCEPT AND EPIDEMIOLOGY

Daniel Abehsera[1,*], MD, PhD
and Andrés C. López[1], MD, PhD
[1]Obstetrics and Gynecology Department,
Quirónsalud Hospital, Málaga, Spain

1. INTRODUCTION

Pelvic inflammatory disease (PID) covers a broad spectrum of infectious processes that affect the different structures of the internal genital tract of women. It is important to bear in mind that depending on the structures affected, the symptoms may vary, although pelvic pain will always be present in all cases.

It will not always be possible to carry out an etiological diagnosis of PID, since in many cases the germs are difficult to cultivate. In most cases, this requires an empirical antibiotic treatment. For this reason, it is important to know what type of germs are those that produce PID in our

* Corresponding Author's Email: daniel.abehsera@quironsalud.es.

environment, and to know what type of germs tend to occur more frequently depending on the type of patient.

It is important to carry out an early diagnosis and treatment of this disease, since the sequelae are serious, and in many cases its severity depends on the speed of establishment of the treatment. The severity of the PID sequelaes implies that this disease generates a high economic cost, not only in the acute episode, but also in the treatment of the sequelaes in the future.

For all the above, it is essential to be clear about the concept of what is a PID, as well as the type of patient who suffers from the disease.

2. CONCEPT

PID is defined as inflammation and infection of the upper genital tract in women. It usually affects the fallopian tubes, ovaries, and adjacent structures; and comprises a variety of inflammatory disorders of the upper genital tract including combinations of endometritis, salpingitis, tube - ovarian abscesses (TOA) and pelviperitonitis. In its origin could be involved germs transmitted by sexual contagion, especially *Neisseria gonorrhoeae* and *Chlamydia trachomatis*, although the usual microorganisms of the vaginal flora may also be involved in its development. The infection by these germs modifies the microbiological balance of the vagina, making it possible to proliferate some strains (gram negative and positive facultative and anaerobic germs) that are responsible for the formation of abscesses at the tubal level [1].

At present, infections associated with pregnancy (septic abortion, intra-amniotic infection, puerperal infection) or those resulting from invasive procedures of the upper genital tract that are considered postoperative infections, are excluded (although they have the same symptomatology and the sequels are analogous). Genital tuberculosis is also excluded, although it may produce the same sequels, it is a different entity [1].

Two phases of the disease can be distinguished. In the first, inflammation of the soft tissues of the pelvis occurs with the involvement of facultative aerobic germs. In the second phase, intra-abdominal abscesses can be formed with the involvement of anaerobic germs [1].

2.1. Endometritis

The presence of plasma cells and neutrophils is observed, and it does not have specific histological characteristics. You can see images more variegated than the classical premenstrual physiological leukocyte infiltration of the endometrium.

Occasionally there may be focal lesions (endometritis on plaques). Healing and repair usually occur without sequels, favored by periodic menstrual desquamation [2].

2.2. Salpingitis

Salpingitis is the fundamental lesion that never fails. In the precocious or mild forms, the tube appears edematous and slightly reddened with the congestive mucosa; purulent fluid can flow through the tubal ostium, but the mobility of the tube is preserved. In moderate cases the mobility of the tube is limited, the fimbrias agglutinate, and the tube tends to adhere to neighboring structures [2].

Salpingitis may only affect the tube on one side or it can be bilateral and may be limited to the organ or coexist with an inflammation of the ovary. If the process is of short duration (acute salpingitis), an infiltrate of neutrophil polymorphonuclear will predominate in the wall of the organ; whereas if the process is of long duration (chronic salpingitis), it will proceed with fibrosis and adhesions. In cases of chronic salpingitis, repeated acute outbreaks usually occur, and distal tubal obstruction and accumulation of fluid inside the organ (pyosalpinx - hydrosalpinx) may occur [3].

2.3. Tube - Ovarian Abscesses and Pelviperitonitis

In severe forms of PID, the entire pelvic cavity appears occluded by an inflammatory mass, there is destruction of the normal anatomy, and formation of TOAs; whose rupture can trigger generalized peritonitis. In any case, the most frequent thing is that the process is limited to the pelvic cavity (pelvic - peritonitis) [2].

The ovary can be affected by adhesion of the inflammatory mass to its surface. The involvement of the ovarian parenchyma is very rare. The TOA formation occurs when a cavity develops in the adherence between the tube and the ovary. These abscesses can involve other organs (for example the bowel), leading to an adherent blockage of all pelvic structures [2].

3. Epidemiology

In the developed countries we find a decrease in the prevalence of this disease, with fewer cases diagnosed both in the hospital setting and in the outpatient setting (Figure 1). Several factors may be contributing to the decrease in PID rates, including increases in the coverage of chlamydia and gonorrhea screening, more sensitive diagnostic technologies, and the availability of single dose therapies that increase adherence to treatment [4].

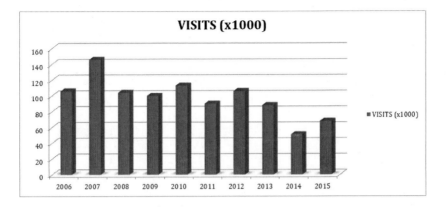

Figure 1. Initial Visits to Physicians' Offices with diagnosis of pelvic inflammatory disease among Women Aged 15–44 Years, United States, 2006-2015 (Centers for Disease Control and Prevention (CDC). Pelvic Inflammatory Disease (PID). http://www.cdc.gov/std/pid/stats.htm (Accessed on May 30, 2018)).

The average cost per patient diagnosed with PID, aged between 20 and 24 years, is $2150. The average lifetime cost for women who developed major complications range between $1270 and $6840, depending on the specific complication (e.g., $6840 in case of ectopic pregnancy). The average cost per person for life for a woman with PID range between $1060 and $3180 [5].

When discussing the epidemiology of PID, it is necessary to differentiate between different age groups, since the presence of the various forms of this disease is influenced by the sexual activity of the patients. It is also interesting to perform an individualized analysis based on the germs involved. The fact that it is not a notifiable disease makes the assessment of epidemiological data very complicated.

3.1. Pelvic Inflammatory Disease in Sexually Experienced Women of Reproductive Age

Data collected in 1444 American women between 18 and 44 years (table 1), showed a prevalence of the PID of 4'4%.

Table 1. Prevalence of pelvic inflammatory disease in sexually experienced women of reproductive age

Higher in those patients who had previously a diagnosis of sexually transmitted infection	Lower in those patients who had not previously a diagnosis of sexually transmitted infection
Higher in those patients with sexual debut before age 12	Lower in those patients with sexual debut after age 18
Higher in those patients who had more than 10 sexual partners	Lower in those patients who had only one sexual partner
Higher in homosexual and bisexual patients	Lower in heterosexual patients

Kreisel, K., Torrone, E., Bernstein, K., Hong, J., Gorwitz, R. 2017. "Prevalence of Pelvic Inflammatory Disease in Sexually Experienced Women of Reproductive Age – United States, 2013-2014". MMWR. Morbidity and mortality weekly report; 27;66(3):80 - 83.

Among the PID cases, it was observed that the prevalence was higher (the triple) in those patients who had previously a diagnosis of sexually transmitted infection (STI). These data showed differences in the prevalence of the disease depending on the age of sexual debut, so that patients with sexual debut before age 12 had 8 times higher prevalence than those with sexual debut after 18 years old. In the same way, the prevalence of PID was 3 times higher in those patients who had more than 10 sexual partners, compared to those who had only one sexual partner.

There were also differences in the prevalence of PID according to sexual orientation, being the half in heterosexual patients versus homosexual and bisexual patients [6].

According to these data, the cases of PID in patients of reproductive age are directly related to the lifestyle of the patients (number of sexual partners, coexistence of other sexually transmitted infections, age of onset of sexual intercourse, etc.).

3.2. Pelvic Inflammatory Disease in Postmenopausal Women

It is estimated that less than 2% of patients admitted to hospitals for salpingitis and TOA are postmenopausal. However, according to data obtained from a study conducted in India on 530 postmenopausal patients, the PID has prevalence in this age group of 11.55%. Therefore, the prevalence of the disease in this age group is not clear. In any case, a series of risk factors (Table 2) have been observed in postmenopausal women that favor the development of a PID [7].Analyzing these data, it can be asserted that PID is a rare disease in postmenopausal women. In addition, STI seem to take a back seat in these cases.

3.3. Pelvic Inflammatory Disease in Paediatrics Patients

PID is also present in the pediatric age. In a US study conducted on 10324 pediatric emergencies in patients between 13 and 19 years of age, a prevalence of the disease of 1.4% was found.

Table 2. Risk factors for pelvic inflammatory disease in postmenopausal women

Higher prevalence increasing with age
Parity is not a risk factor
Higher prevalence in patients with multiple sexual contacts
Higher prevalence in patients with pelvic organ prolapse
Higher prevalence in patients with bacterial vaginosis
Chronic disease is not a risk factor
Smoking is not a risk factor

Khan, S., Ansari, M. A., Vasenwala, S. M., Mohsin, Z. 2017. "A Community Based Study on Pelvic Inflammatory Disease in Postmenopausal Females: Microbiological Spectrum and Socio-Demographic Correlates". Journal of clinical and diagnostic research: JCDR; 11(3):LC05-LC10.

PID was diagnosed in 9.2% of female adolescents with a chief complaint of abdominal and/or pelvic pain. The presence of STI was detected in less than half of the cases, being the germ most frequently detected *Chlamydia trachomatis*. Most of the cases did not require hospital admission, and they were resolved with antibiotic treatment administered orally [8]. Therefore, the PID is a table to take into account in pediatric age, and as in the case of women of reproductive age, it is directly related to STI. The behavior of the disease seems to be milder than in other stages of life.

3.4. Gonococcal and Chlamydial Pelvic Inflammatory Disease

Classically, a causal relationship has been established between PID and infection with gonorrhea and chlamydia; however, there are probably profound geographical differences in the prevalence of these germs in cases of PID. The median age of patients was 20 years. The most common patient complaint was abnormal vaginal discharge, followed by abdominal pain and/or dyspareunia and dysuria. On clinical examination, more than one third of patients had mucopurulent cervical discharge, and 30 cases had a friable cervix. Seventy-seven patients had a swab for wet mount taken at the time of diagnosis. There were no cases of HIV coinfection [9].

Probably both chlamydia and gonorrhea play an important role in the genesis of PID in women of reproductive age, occupying a more secondary place in postmenopausal women.

3.5. The Role of Mycoplasma Genitalium

A meta-analysis of studies in women has demonstrated a significant association of *Mycoplasma genitalium* with pelvic inflammatory disease.

Seña et al. found a prevalence of *Mycoplasma genitalium* was almost twice that of *Chamydia trachomatis* and 5 times that of *Neisseria gonorrhoeae* in their population, and *Mycoplasma genitalium* coinfected 24% - 30% of women who had either chlamydial or gonococcal infections [10].

Based on these data, it seems advisable to perform the detection test of genital mycoplasmas in cases of suspected PID. Probably many of the PID cases that remain without detection of causative agent, are due to the infection by Mycoplasma genitalium.

REFERENCES

[1]   Xercavins, Jordi. 2004. *Enfermedad inflamatoria pélvica. [Pelvic Inflammatory Disease]*. Madrid: Meditex. (Xercavins 2004, 107).

[2]   Usandizaga, José A., and de la Fuente, Pedro. 1998. *Tratado de Obstetricia y Ginecología [Treaty of Obstetrics and Gynecology], Vol II*. Madrid: McGraw-Hill (Usandizaga and de la Fuente 1998, 224 – 225).

[3]   Grasés, Pedro J. 2003. *Patología Ginecológica [Gynecological pathology]*. Barcelona: Masson (Grasés 2003, 112).

[4]   Centers for Disease Control and Prevention (CDC). *Pelvic Inflammatory Disease* (PID). http://www.cdc.gov/std/pid/stats.htm (Accessed on May 30, 2018).

[5]   Yeh, J. M., Hook, E. W. 3rd, Goldie, S. J. 2003. "A refined estimate of the average lifetime cost of pelvic inflammatory disease". *Sexually transmitted diseases*, 30(5):369 - 78.

[6]   Kreisel, K., Torrone, E., Bernstein, K., Hong, J., Gorwitz, R. 2017. "Prevalence of Pelvic Inflammatory Disease in Sexually Experienced Women of Reproductive Age – United States, 2013-2014". *MMWR. Morbidity and mortality weekly report*, 27; 66(3): 80 - 83.

[7]   Khan, S., Ansari, M. A., Vasenwala, S. M., Mohsin, Z. 2017. "A Community Based Study on Pelvic Inflammatory Disease in Postmenopausal Females: Microbiological Spectrum and Socio-Demographic Correlates". *Journal of clinical and diagnostic research: JCDR*, 11(3):LC05-LC10.

[8]   Solomon, M., Tuchman, L., Hayes, K., Badolato, G., Goyal, M. K. 2017. "Pelvic Inflammatory Disease in a Pediatric Emergency Department: Epidemiology and Treatment". *Pediatric emergency care*, Article in press.

[9]   Chen, J. Z., Gratrix, J., Smyczek, P., Parker, P., Read, R., Singh, A. E. 2018. "Gonococcal and Chlamydial Cases of Pelvic Inflammatory Disease at 2 Canadian Sexually Transmitted Infection Clinics, 2004 to 2014: A Retrospective Cross-sectional Review". *Sexually transmitted diseases*, 45(4):280 - 282.

[10] Seña, A. C., Lee, J. Y., Schwebke, J., Philip, S. S., Wiesenfeld, H. C., Rompalo, A. M., Cook, R. L., Hobbs, M. M. 2018. "A silent epidemic: the prevalence, incidence and persistence of Mycoplasma genitalium among young, asymptomatic high-risk women in the United States". *Clinical infectious diseases: an official publication of the Infectious Diseases Society of America*, Article in press.

In: Pelvic Inflammatory Disease
Editor: Daniel Abehsera

ISBN: 978-1-53615-193-0
© 2019 Nova Science Publishers, Inc.

Chapter 2

CLINICAL MANIFESTATIONS AND DIAGNOSTIC CRITERIA

Laura Baños[1],, MD and Jessica Martín[1], MD*
[1]Obstetrics and Gynecology Department,
Quirónsalud Hospital, Málaga, Spain

1. INTRODUCTION

Pelvic inflammatory disease (PID) has a wide spectrum of symptoms and clinical manifestations that can cause the diagnosis to be delayed or confused with other diseases with similar symptoms if there is no obvious pelvic symptomatology. This pathology can affect one or more of the following anatomical situations: endometritis, salpingitis, oophoritis, pelvic peritonitis, and perihepatitis. The diagnosis of PID is not always easy, so we are going to summarize the most frequent clinical manifestations and the criteria on which we have to base ourselves to make an accurate diagnosis.

* Corresponding Author's Email: laura.banos@quironsalud.es.

This disease can be associated with future complications, so a diagnosis is important in the early stages to start treatment as soon as possible. We will differentiate the need for outpatient or inpatient treatment according to the severity of the condition. There is no a single diagnostic gold standard for PID because of the multiple infection variants. Clinical diagnosis remains the most important practical approach.

2. CLINICAL MANIFESTATIONS

PID is particularly common among sexually active young and adolescent women. The majority of PID cases, around 85%, are caused by sexually transmitted infections (STI). The remaining 15% may be caused by germs associated with the intestinal tract or respiratory infections that have colonized the lower genital tract [1].

Any sexually active female is at risk of a STI associated with PID, but it is logical to think that the greater number of sexual partners a woman has the greater the risk of infection. The highest risk of PID is in women who undergo instrumentation of the cervix. Older women present less commonly with PID, but when they do, the cause is more likely to be non-STI related [1, 2].

The clinical spectrum of this disease varies from the asymptomatic process to the vital commitment. The most frequent clinical condition of PID is a patient with pelvic pain and scarce affectation of the general state since only a small percentage of patients present the severe pelviperitonitis forms. Infection of the lower genital tract that precedes the clinical picture may go unnoticed or cause only slight genitourinary discomfort, since cervicitis is usually asymptomatic or produces leucorrhoea. The appearance of pelvic pain is the first symptom indicative of an ascending infection and is usually located in the lower abdomen (hypogastrium or with bilateral extension to both iliac fossae) begin subacute, persistent and not very intense [3].

We will divide the clinical forms of PID according to the presentation in acute, subacute and chronic. We understand acute as a presentation of less than 30 days and chronic as more than 30 days [4].

The symptoms associated with acute PID include lower abdominal or pelvic pain, pelvic organ tenderness and inflammation of the genital tract. Pain is the most common symptom in women with PID. Pelvic tenderness of any kind has high sensitivity (> 95%) for PID, but it has poor specificity [1]. Pain is variable in each patient, from intense pain to mild pain. It is typical that pain increases with coitus, sudden movements or after menstruation [2]. The clinical manifestations of the disease can vary from the silent form to sepsis with severe involvement of the general state. Most of PIDs are a mild to moderate presentation of the disease, and it is not frequent to develop severe manifestations. Other symptoms associated are abnormal vaginal discharge (Image 1), intermenstrual or postcoital bleeding, dyspareunia, and dysuria. This abnormal bleeding appears in approximately one third of patients [4].

According to some authors, the appearance of metrorrhagia in a sexually active young woman who is not a user of hormonal contraception means we must discard genital infection (endometritis) as a possibility especially if it coexists with other genitourinary symptoms.

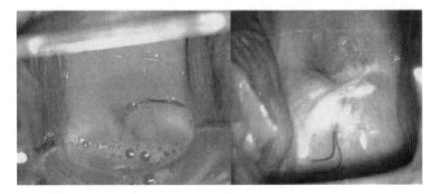

Image 1. Abnormal vaginal discharge in patient with intrauterine device.

Dysuria can occur in 20% of cases associated with the detection of the same germs in urinary tract [5].

On physical examination, most women have abdominal tenderness on palpation, greatest in the lower quadrants, which may or may not be symmetrical. As previously explained, fever and other systemic features are usually limited to women with more severe PIDs. [4].

The most characteristic symptoms are pain on mobilization of the cervix and adnexal tenderness during bimanual pelvic examination. Purulent endocervical discharge is also common [2]. Leucorrhoea occurs approximately in half of the cases (Image 2), often preceding the clinical manifestation of acute PID, as the first manifestation of cervicitis and dyspareunia [3]. The abdominal pain is usually bilateral but on exam we can see pain being unilateral because of a tubo-ovarian abscess.

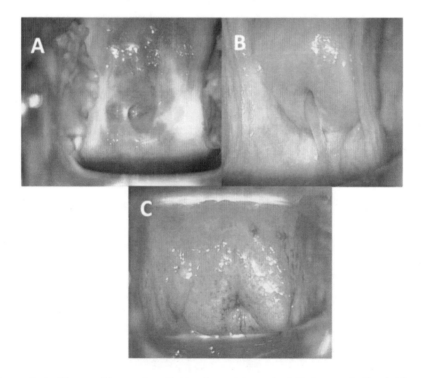

Image 2. A: Abnormal leucorrhea. B: Purulent endocervical discharge. C: Cervicitis.

This is an inflammatory mass involving a fallopian tube, an ovary and any other pelvic organs. Tubo-ovarian abscesses are usually a complication of PID [6].

Other severe complication is perihepatitis (Fitz-Hugh-Curtis syndrome). Occasionally, right-upper-quadrant pain suggestive of inflammation and adhesion formation in the liver capsule can accompany PID [1]. The incidence of Fitz-Hugh-Curtis syndrome depends on the criteria we use for the diagnosis. There may be an asymptomatic patient with evidence of perihepatic adhesions seen at laparoscopy and on the other hand a patient with PID and right-upper quadrant pain without evidence of signs of perihepatitis [7]. This pain appears in 1 - 10% of cases of acute PIDs, may reflect perihepatitis [3]. The diagnosis of Fitz-Hugh-Curtis syndrome can be difficult, as its symptoms and physical findings can mimic those of many other diseases like cholelithiasis, cholecystitis, pleurisy or pneumonia [7]. Perihepatitis can be definitively distinguished from other causes of right upper quadrant pain only by directly visualizing the liver. Perihepatitis is inflammation of the liver capsule and peritoneal surfaces of the anterior right upper quadrant. On physical examination, we can see marked tenderness in the right upper quadrant. Laparoscopy shows the so-called "violin strings" adhesions, caused by a patchy purulent and fibrinous exudate [8]. Using clinical and laparoscopic criteria the rate of coincident of perihepatitis and PID was similar, between 12 to 13.8%. The diagnosis of the syndrome is more frequent in women with intrauterine contraceptive device (IUD) who had insertion in the last 6 weeks compared to those who had it for a longer time [7]. In PID origin germs transmitted by sexual contagion are involved, especially Neisseria gonorrhoeae and Chlamydia trachomatis, although the usual microorganisms of the vaginal flora may also be involved in their development. These sexually transmitted agents ascend into the upper genital tract, distinguishing it from pelvic infections caused by transcervical medical procedures (IUD), pregnancy and other primary abdominal processes that can extend to pelvic organs [3]. The pathogenesis of Fitz-Hugh-Curtis syndrome is understood. It may result from direct, hematogenous, or lymphatic infection of the liver capsule and related structures [7].

Due to the possible complications, a prompt diagnosis and treatment to reduce the risk of both short- and long-term complications is very important [9].

3. CLINICAL STAGING

In order to deal with the therapeutic problem, Monif (1982) developed the Gainesville clinical classification of the disease divided into four stages as we can see in table 1. Most patients admitted in gynecological ward belong to stage II [10].

Table 1. Gainesville clinical classification of the pelvic inflammatory disease

Stage	Clinical findings	Treatment
I	Salpingitis without peritonitis	Patients can be treated on an outpatient basis
II	Salpingitis with peritonitis	Requiring hospitalization and intravenous antibiotic therapy
III	PID with a pelvic mass	Hospitalization and intravenous therapy
IV	Tubo-ovarian abscess which has ruptured	Hospitalization and intravenous therapy

Monif GR. (1982). Clinical staging of acute bacterial salpingitis and its therapeutic ramifications. American journal of obstetrics and gynecology.1;143(5):489 - 95.

4. EVALUATION

PID should be suspected in any young or sexually active female patient who presents with lower abdominal pain and pelvic discomfort [11]. The genital examination should be initiated by an inspection of external genital area, enabling the detection of STIs and or stigmas (ulcers, vesicles, condylomas). Using speculcopy, we evaluate the vagina and cervix, for signs of inflammation, the presence of leucorrhoea and, occasionally, discharge of exudate through the external cervical orifice (spontaneously or after slightly pressing with the speculum), proceeding at that moment to collect endocervical specimens and which will serve to perform gram stains, fresh smears and microbiological cultures (Image 3) [3].

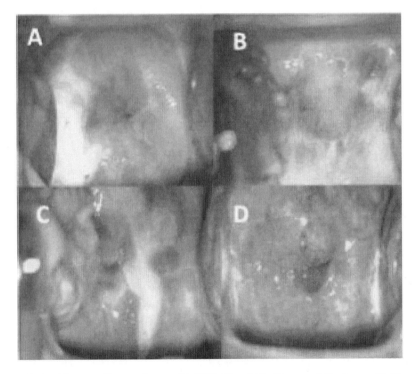

Image 3. A: Abnormal leucorrhoea with IUD. B and C: Abnormal discharge. D: Cervix with signs of inflammation.

Abdominovaginal combined exploration may cause pain to the cervical mobilization and pressure of the Douglas although sometimes we will not obtain information from the examination due to the muscular defense that the patient can offer. The palpation of the adnexal area is painful and can be felt thickened, fixed and very sensitive to the pressure exerted on them.

In cases in which the process has evolved to a tubo-ovarian abscess, it will be possible to delimit in one or both of the adnexal areas a poorly defined irregular tumor, close to the uterus, which is painful and totally fixed [3].

Based on the clinical history and the exploration we can make a diagnosis of a suspicion of a PID. Although laboratory testing is also done at the initial evaluation of all patients with suspected PID, empiric treatment should not be delayed while awaiting results of these supportive tests [2].

Additional diagnostic and imaging tests will be covered in another chapter.

5. DIAGNOSTIC CRITERIA

The clinical diagnosis of PID is based on doing a thorough physical exam. With bimanual examination, we can show pelvic organ tenderness, as indicated by cervical motion tenderness, adnexal tenderness, or uterine compression tenderness.

This exam, in conjunction with signs of lower genital tract inflammation, guides us towards the diagnosis of PID [8].

Part of the signs of lower genital tract inflammation are cervical mucopus (an exudate from the endocervix or as yellow or green mucus), cervical friability (easily induced columnar epithelial bleeding) or increased numbers of white cells observed on the saline microscopic examination of vaginal secretions [1].

Table 2. Diagnostic criteria of pelvic inflammatory disease

Hager criteria (1983)	CDC criteria (2002)
Minimum criteria (all) Abdominal pain with or without signs of peritoneal irritation Pain with cervical motion Pain palpation adnexal área, And one of the following: Fever ≥ 38°C Leukocytosis > 10.500 / mm3 Purulent fluid in vaginal discharge (with leukocytes and bacteria) VSG > 15 (1st hour) Inflammatory mass by palpation and/or ultrasound Presence of de *Neisseria gonorrhoeae* y/o *Chlamydia trachomatis* in endocérvix	**Minimum criteria** Uterine or adnexal pain Pain with cervical motion **Additional criteria to increase specificity** Leukocytosis in the smear in fresh vaginal Abnormal vaginal and/or cervical leukorrhea Fever > 38,3° C Increase in VSG or C-reactive protein Laboratory evidence of Neisseria gonorrhoeae and/or Chlamydia trachomatis in endocervix

Xercavins Montosa, J. (2004). Enfermedad inflamatoria pélvica. Documentos de consenso SEGO. 105 - 134.

For the clinical diagnosis, the Hager criteria of 1983 have been used classically, requiring the existence of abdominal palpation pain, pain to the cervical mobilization and pain to the adnexal examination (Table 2) and any of the following: leukocytosis, erythrosedimentation greater than 15 in the 1st hour, fever higher than 38°C, obtaining purulent fluid from the Douglas pouch, pelvic echographic abscess and/or detection of Neisseria gonorrhoeae and/or Chlamydia trachomatis in the endocervical study [3]. The Centers for Disease Control and Prevention (CDC) in 2015 considers that the pain must be present in the three locations to determine the diagnosis dangerously decreases sensitivity, so it recommends that new criteria according to which the empirical treatment should be initiated (Table 2) in the presence of any of the following signs: pain to the uterine mobilization, adnexal or pain to the cervical mobilization. The sensitivity is still low, 65 - 90%, but the potential sequelae of the disease justify the initiation of antibiotic therapy [2, 12].

In our service we follow a diagnostic protocol according to which we classify the patient based on the need for outpatient treatment or hospitalization. In order to classify the patients, we first performed an analytical test with a complete blood count, a C-reactive protein, a pregnancy test, and an examination with vaginal cultures and ultrasound.

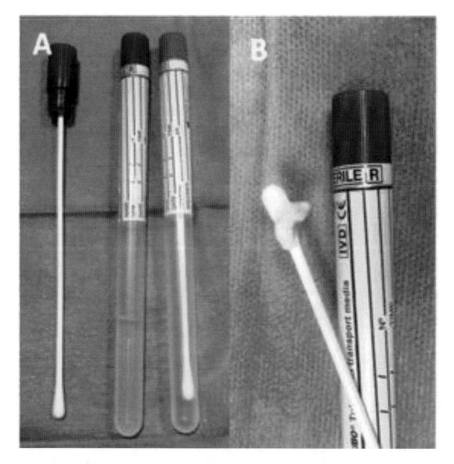

Image 4. A: Swabs for sampling. B: Pathological exudate simple.

Within the protocol we use, we take several crop samples for the diagnosis.

A sample of vaginal leucorrhoea is taken from the endocervix, another from the urethra whenever there is a urethritis clinic and a sample without medium for the study of Chlamydia trachomatis (Images 4 and 5).

The classification of the need for outpatient or hospital treatment is based on clinical, analytical, and physical examination criteria. In table 3 are shown the different criteria between both treatments.

According to the protocol, in that IUD carrier patient we recommend the withdrawal and sending of the device to the laboratory for microbiological culture.

The different treatment options will be explained in the corresponding chapter.

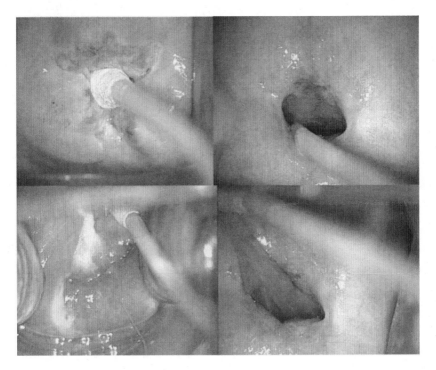

Image 5. Vaginal cultures.

Laura Baños and Jessica Martín

Table 3. Criteria for ambulatory treatment vs hospital treatment

Outpatient treatment	Hospital Treatment
Fever < 38,3°C	Uncertain diagnosis that does not exclude the possibility of surgery such as
Leukocytes < 11000 / mm³	appendicitis or ectopic pregnancy
	Suspicion of pelvic abscess
No evidence of peritonitis	Pregnancy
	Teen patient
Intestinal noises present	Patient with human immunodeficiency virus
Oral tolerance	Concomitance with serious illness
	Intrauterine device
	Recent uterine instrumentation

REFERENCES

[1] Brunham, R. C., Gottlieb, S. L., Paavonen, J. 2015. "Pelvic inflammatory disease". *New England Journal of Medicine*, 372 (21), 2039 - 2048.

[2] Ross, J., Judlin, P., Jensen, J. 2014. "2012 European guideline for the management of pelvic inflammatory disease". *International journal of STD & AIDS*, 25:1.

[3] Xercavins, J. 2004. *Enfermedad inflamatoria pélvica, Documentos de consenso SEGO* [*Pelvic inflammatory disease, SEGO Consensus documents*], 105 - 134.

[4] Wiesenfeld, H. C., Sweet, R. L., Ness, R. B., Krohn, M. A., Amortegui, A. J., Hillier, S. L. 2005. "Comparison of acute and subclinical pelvic inflammatory disease". *Sexually Transmitted Diseases*, 32:400 - 405.

[5] Eckert, L. O., Hawes, S. E., Wolner-Hanssen, P. K., Kiviat, N. B., Wasserheit, J. N., Paavonen, J. A., Eschenbach, D. A., Holmes, K. K. 2002. "Endometritis: The clinical–pathologic syndrome". *American Journal of Obstetrics and Gynecology,* 186:690 - 695.

[6] Lareau, S. M., Beigi, R. H. 2008. "Pelvic inflammatory disease and tubo-ovarian abscess". *Infectious Disease Clinics of North America*, 22:693.

[7] Peter, N. G., Clark, L. R., Jaeger, R. J. 2004. "Fitz-Hugh-Curtis syndrome: A diagnosis to consider in women with right upper quadrant pain". *Cleveland Clinic Journal of Medicine*, 71:3. 233 - 239.

[8] Ross, J., Cole, M., Evans, C., Lyons, D., Dean, G., Cousins, D. (2018). *United Kingdom National Guideline for the Management of Pelvic Inflammatory Disease.* URL: http://www.bashh.org/ guidelines.

[9] Soper, D. E. 2010. "Pelvic inflammatory disease". *Obstetrict and Gynecology,* 116:419.

[10] Muylder, X. 1986. "Treatment of acute pelvic inflammatory disease with penicillin and chloramphenicol in a developing country". *Annales de la Société Belge de Médecine Tropicale*, 66, 177 - 182.

[11] Kreisel, K., Torrone, E., Bernstein, K., Hong, J., Gorwitz, R. 2017. "Prevalence of Pelvic Inflammatory Disease in Sexually Experienced Women of Reproductive Age. United States, 2013-2014". MMWR. *Morbidity and mortality weekly report*, 27; 66(3):80 - 83.

[12] Workowski, K. A., Bolan, G. A., Centers for Disease Control and Prevention. 2015. "Sexually transmitted diseases treatment guidelines". *Clinical Infectious Diseases*, 64(33), 924.

In: Pelvic Inflammatory Disease   ISBN: 978-1-53615-193-0
Editor: Daniel Abehsera   © 2019 Nova Science Publishers, Inc.

Chapter 3

MICROBIOLOGY OF THE PELVIC INFLAMMATORY DISEASE: MOLECULAR BIOLOGY TECHNIQUES

Laura López[1,*], MD and Paula Chamocho[1], MD
[1]Obstetrics and Gynecology Department,
Quirónsalud Hospital, Málaga, Spain

1. INTRODUCTION

In this chapter we will specify the most frequent agents involved in pelvic inflammatory disease and available diagnostic methods. *Neisseria gonorrhoeae and Chlamydia trachomatis* are the most commonly identified pathogens in pelvic inflammatory disease (PID) Among Sexually Active Premenopausal Females. *Mycoplasma Genitalium* Is Also Likely To Be A Cause In The Premenopausal Group. *Echerichia Coli* And Colonic Anaerobes May Be Responsible For The Rare cases of

---

* Corresponding Author's Email: lvlopez.mlg@quironsalud.es.

PID seen in postmenopausal women. Very rare pathogens identified include *Mycobacterium tuberculosis* and the agents of actinomycosis. However, in most cases, the precise microbial etiology of PID is unknown. Regardless of the initiating pathogen, PID is clinically considered a mixed infection [1].

2. MICROBIOLOGY OF THE PELVIC INFLAMMATORY DISEASE

2.1. Chlamydia Trachomatis

Chlamydia trachomatis is a small gram-negative bacterium that is an obligate intracellular parasite. It has a distinct life-cycle consisting of two major phases [2]:

- The small elementary bodies attach and penetrate into cells, changing into the metabolically active form, called the reticulate body, within six to eight hours. These forms create large inclusions within cells.
- The reticulate bodies then reorganize into small elementary bodies, and within two to three days the cell ruptures, releasing newly formed elementary bodies. Release of the elementary bodies initiates the replicative process, since this is the form that can infect new epithelial cells. The long growth cycle explains why treatment with agents with long half-lives or a prolonged course of antibiotics is necessary to eradicate infection.

Genital infection with *Chlamydia trachomatis* is the most common bacterial sexually transmitted infection, especially among young women [2] Figure 1.

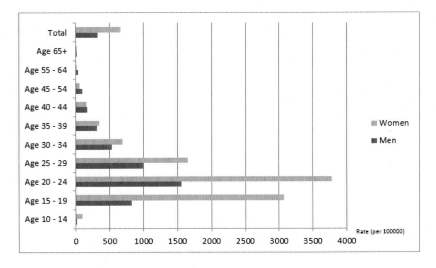

Figure 1. Chlamydia rates by age and sex in the Unites States in 2016 (Marrazzo J. 2016. "Treatment of Chlamydia Trachomatis infection". URL: https://www.uptodate.com).

Because the majority (~70 - 80%) of lower genital tract *Chlamydia trachomatis* infections in women remains asymptomatic, patients may not seek testing for care. If untreated, genital chlamydial infection can ascend to the upper genital tract, leading to serious complications such as PID, tubal factor infertility and ectopic pregnancy [3].

Several trials have suggested that screening young women for chlamydia reduces the rate of subsequent PID, although some limitations reduce certainty about the findings [3, 4]. As an example, in a trial of female college students in London, all participants provided vaginal swabs at study entry and were then randomly assigned to screening (in which the samples were tested for chlamydia and those with positive tests were treated) or control (in which the samples were stored and analyzed at the end of the study) [5]. Among those with chlamydia at baseline, 1 of 63 in the intervention group versus 7 of 74 in the control group developed PID (RR 0.17, 95% CI 0.03 - 1.01). However, 30 of the 38 cases of PID observed in the study occurred in participants with negative baseline chlamydia, and 10 of those cases were documented to be associated with chlamydia. These findings indicate the importance of ongoing chlamydial transmission and the need for repeated screening over time in at-risk individuals [5].

2.2. Neisseria Gonorrhoeae

Gonorrhea is an ancient human disease, with references to its symptoms found in the Old Testament of the Bible (Leviticus 15:1-3) [6]. The gram-negative pathogen Neisseria gonorrhoeae is the causative agent of the sexually transmitted infection gonorrhea, which affects approximately 100 million people globally. Disease in women is associated with cervicitis which can be asymptomatic leading to continued transmission between sex partners. Moreover, a subset of women with gonococcal infection will develop upper genital tract disease, which can lead to pelvic inflammatory disease, ectopic pregnancy, and tubal infertility [7].

Neonatal health is also detrimentally affected by gonococcus infection, as this pathogen can cause a sight-threatening conjunctivitis in infants born to infected mothers [8].

2.3. Mycoplasma Genitalium

Over 200 named *Mycoplasma* species exist. However, only about six species, five of which inhabit the genitourinary tract, are established or presumed human pathogens. Mycoplasmas that are thought to cause disease in humans include *Mycoplasma pneumoniae*, *Mycoplasma hominis*, *Mycoplasma genitalium*, *Mycoplasma fermentans* (incognitus strain), *Ureaplasma urealyticum*, and *Ureaplasma parvum* [5]. Mycoplasmas and ureaplasmas are the smallest free-living organisms. Because they lack a cell wall, neither mycoplasmas nor ureaplasmas can be visualized by Gram stain.

In order to culture these organisms, specialized media containing animal serum is required *Mycoplasma hominis* has been associated with chorioamnionitis. A possible association with PID is less well established. Non-genitourinary tract infections that have been reported include upper and lower respiratory infections, central nervous system infections, neonatal bacteremia and meningoencephalitis, and others. *Ureaplasma* spp have been linked to chorioamnionitis, postpartum and postabortal fever, and pneumonia, bacteremia, and abscesses in neonates. There is controversy about a possible association between *Ureaplasma* spp and bronchopulmonary dysplasia [9].

2.4. Bacterial Vaginosis

Is the most common microbiological disorder affecting the vaginal flora and is often accompanied by pathologic malodorous discharge. However, bacterial vaginosis can also be asymptomatic. There are no precise figures on the prevalence. The reported prevalence in Europe is between 5 and more than 30% of the population of gynecological patients; the reported incidence in pregnant women is between 7 and 22% [10].

Bacterial vaginosis, vaginitis or cervicitis diagnosed using any of the methods with lower abdominal pain, cervical motion tenderness or tenderness of the uterus and/or of the adnexa on pressure suggest acute PID [10].

2.5. Other Initiating Pathogens

Other agents that initiate PID, while almost certainly sexually transmitted and probably infectious, remain obscure. Using molecular amplification with generic primers, a number of novel bacteria have been identified in the fallopian tubes of women with PID, including Atopobium, Sneathia, and Leptotrichia. The role of these and other anaerobic bacteria in the pathogenesis of PID remains to be proven [8].

2.6. Mixed Infection

Some studies found that, among cases of PID initiated by Neiseria gonorrhoeae, a mixed polymicrobial infection was seen in approximately 35 percent of cases. Other studies, which employed particularly stringent microbiologic techniques, identified other organisms in more than 50 percent of patients with gonococcal PID [9].

3. MOLECULAR BIOLOGY TECHNIQUES

According to the protocol followed in our center, the taking of tests should be as follows:

- Vaginal sampling whenever there is leucorrhea.
- Associate endocervical sampling always.
- Urethral sampling if there are signs of urethritis.
- Sample taking without medium for chlamydia trachomatis.

3.1. Molecular Diagnostics for *Chlamydia Trachomatis*

Diagnostic techniques include nucleic acid amplification (NAAT), culture, antigen detection and genetic probes; microscopy is not useful for the diagnosis of chlamydia. Because of superior sensitivity and specificity, NAAT is the diagnostic technique of choice, where available. With this technique, noninvasive screening options, such as first-catch urine testing or self-collected vaginal swabs, are possible and have become the diagnostic approach of choice for chlamydial (and gonococcal) infections. However, for women presenting with symptomatic cervicitis that undergo a speculum exam, or for high-risk women undergoing routine Pap smear, NAAT can be performed on either endocervical or vaginal swabs.

Swabs should have a plastic or wire shaft and rayon, dacron, or cytobrush tip, as other materials may be inhibitory to the organism [11].

- **Nucleic acid amplification:** NAAT methodology consists of amplifying *Chlamydia trachomatis* DNA or RNA sequences using polymerase chain reaction (PCR), transcription-mediated amplification (TMA), or strand displacement amplification (SDA). These sensitive and specific tests have become the "gold standard", and are the preferred diagnostic method, if available [11].

- **Test performance by specimen**: A major advantage of NAATs is their excellent performance on specimens that can be collected without having to perform a pelvic examination in women or obtain a urethral swab in men. In fact, in women, a swab of vaginal fluid is the preferred approach for diagnosing chlamydial infection, as this specimen provides the highest sensitivity. First-catch urine submitted for NAAT should be collected from the initial stream (approximately the first 10mL) without pre-cleansing of the genital areas. Ideally, the patient should not have voided in the two hours prior to specimen collection. The performance of these is not affected by the presence of purulent material or blood [12]. A systematic review pooled data from 29 studies to assess the sensitivity and specificity of NAAT for *Chlamydia trachomatis* infection in urine specimens. Summary estimates for sensitivity and specificity were calculated for urine and cervical sampling for three NAAT methods (PCR, TMA, or

SDA). The analysis demonstrated that the sensitivity and specificity of non-invasive testing (urine) was comparable to invasive testing, although more data was available for analysis on PCR testing than the other two methods [13].

- **Rapid tests for Chlamydia:** Although NAAT has replaced culture as the new "gold standard", same-day results have traditionally not been available. These rapid tests provide results within 30 minutes of testing and are less expensive to perform and simple to interpret since testing results are reflected in a test strip color change. An example is the Chlamydia Rapid Test on first-void urine in men. This assay, based on use of a monoclonal antibody to chlamydia lipopolysaccharide, was compared to NAAT (PCR) as a gold standard. The sensitivity, specificity, positive predictive value, and negative predictive value of the Chlamydia Rapid Test was 83 percent, 99 percent, 84 percent, and 98 percent, respectively [14].

- **Culture:** Culture methods are now limited to research and reference laboratories due to the expense and technical expertise required [14].

- **Serology**: *Chalmydia trachomatis* serology (complement fixation titers > 1:64) can support the diagnosis of chlamydia in the appropriate clinical context but is performed infrequently, not standardized, and requires a high level of expertise to interpret [14].

- **Antigen detection:** Antigen detection requires invasive testing using a swab from the cervix or urethra. The sensitivity of this method is 80 to 95 percent compared with culture [14].

- **Genetic probe methods**: Because they do not involve amplification of genetic targets, available genetic probe methods require invasive testing using a direct swab from the cervix or urethra. The sensitivity of this assay is approximately 80 percent compared with culture. The main advantage of these tests is their low cost; however, because their sensitivity is considerably lower than NAAT and because NAAT have become more cost-competitive, these tests are not used as frequently as in the past [14].

3.2. Molecular Diagnostics for *Neisseria Gonorrhoeae*

3.2.1. Advantages of Molecular Diagnostics for Gonorrhoea

There is no commercially available test for gonorrhoea that gives both same-day diagnosis and an antimicrobial susceptibility profile for *Neisseria gonorrhoeae*. But the ability of nucleic acid amplification test (NAAT) to detect tiny amounts of nucleic acid has several advantages over culture for the diagnosis of a *Neisseria gonorrhoeae* infection [15, 16]:

- Specimens for NAATs are easier to transport and store because they do not need the organism to be viable for detection.
- NAATs can be automated and multiplexed detecting both *Chlamydia trachomatis* and *Neisseria gonorrhoeae*, which is useful because both organisms cause similar clinical syndromes [11].
- Analysis can be done on non-invasive self-collected specimens like urine and vaginal swabs. These qualities mean that testing is easier in remote areas and can be extended to groups who were previously hard to reach but at high risk of both infection and antimicrobial resistance (AMR), such as men who have sex with men [15].
- NAATs are more sensitive than culture methods in general and particularly for asymptomatic infections in the pharynx and rectum (although no internationally available commercial NAAT has licensing approval for use on extra-genital samples) [15].

NAATs for *N. gonorrhoeae* diagnosis became available in the early 1990s and are now the most common method used for gonorrhoea diagnosis in many countries, including the United Kingdom and United States. The sharp increase in the number of diagnosed gonorrhoea cases since 2010 is likely to be associated, in part, with both higher numbers of tests and the higher sensitivity of NAAT. In the US, the absolute number of gonorrhoea tests, estimated from data from manufacturers, increased from 2000 to 2004 but the percentage of tests that were done by culture fell [16].

3.2.2. Disadvantages of Molecular Diagnostics for Gonorrhoea

- The main limitation for clinical management is that there is no viable organism so NAATs cannot provide data about minimum inhibitory concentrations for antimicrobials, which guide therapy. All results from NAAT-diagnosed gonococcal infections have to be treated "blind" and commercially available NAATs do not currently detect any antimicrobial resistance determinants, so more NAAT-diagnosed than culture-diagnosed infections will be unnecessarily treated with extended spectrum cephalosporins based regimens [15].
- NAATs encourage over-testing and overtreatment of gonorrhoea. Over-testing is facilitated by simultaneous testing for *Neisseriae gonorrhoeae* on specimens taken for chlamydia screening in populations at low risk of gonorrhoea such as asymptomatic heterosexual adults tested in primary care. In such settings, the predictive value of a positive test for gonorrhoea can be unacceptably low, meaning that most people with a positive test are not infected. Overtreatment will occur if clinicians interpret initial positive gonorrhoea NAAT results as diagnosed infections without supporting information from a sexual history and/or a confirmatory test, as recommended. While some NAATs for *Neisseriae gonorrhoeae* show very high specificity,

their performance is inherently limited by genetic sequence variation between subtypes and cross-reactions with related *Neisseria* species. Overtreatment also has consequences for AMR. Unnecessary use of extended spectrum antimicrobials, such as ceftriaxone, increases the chances that commensal *Neisseria spp.* develops resistance and that resistance determinants will be transferred horizontally to *Neisseriae gonorrhoeae* [11].

- The high cost of NAATs can result in over-testing or under-testing, depending on who has to pay for the test and who makes the profit [11].
- Antimicrobial prescribing policies can also contribute to the emergence of antimicrobial resistance gonorrhoea. Clinical guidelines in Europe and the United States now recommend combination treatment with intramuscular ceftriaxone and oral azithromycin [11, 15-16].

The development of molecular tests to detect gonococcus resistance mutations should become part of the solution. Commercial diagnostics companies should invest more to develop and evaluate NAATs that detect both *Neisseriae gonorrhoeae* and AMR determinants reliably, particularly in resource poor settings [11, 15-16].

3.3. Molecular Biology Techniques of *Mycoplasma Hominis* and *Ureaplasma*

Mycoplasma genitalium is a small bacterium of the mollicutes class with no cell wall and a genome of only 580 kilobases in size. Consequently, it cannot be detected by gram stain and is extremely difficult to culture requiring up to 6 months for growth. Its genome is most similar to Mycoplasma pneumonia. Currently there is no FDA-approved diagnostic test for Mycoplasma genitalium. Given the difficulty with culturing the organism and the lack of standardized serological tests for Mycoplasma genitalium, NAATs in the form of polymerase chain reaction (PCR) assays are almost exclusively carried out for the diagnosis of Mycoplasma genitalium in the research setting. Some PCR assays have demonstrated > 95% specificity and sensitivity. A recent study reported loop-mediated isothermal amplification as a novel NAAT, which has similar sensitivity to a PCR assay [17].

REFERENCES

[1]   Ross, J., Hynes, N. A, Bloom, A. 2017. *"Pelvic inflammatory disease: Pathogenesis, microbiology, and risk factors"*. URL: https://www.uptodate.com.

[2]   Marrazzo, J. 2016. *"Treatment of Chlamydia Trachomatis infection"*. URL: https://www.uptodate.com.

[3]   Scholes, D., Stergachis, A., Heidrich, F. E., Andrilla, H., Holmes, K. K., Stamm, W. E. 1996. "Prevention of pelvic inflammatory disease by screening for cervical chlamydial infection". *The New England journal of medicine,* 23; 334(21):1362 - 6.

[4]   Gottlieb, S. L., Berman, S. M., Low, N. 2010. "Screening and treatment to prevent sequelae in women with Chlamydia trachomatics genital infection: how much do we Know?". *The Journal of infectious diseases*, 201 Suppl. 2:S156.

[5]   Oakeshott, P., Kerry, S., Aghaizu, A., Atherton, H., Hay, S., Taylor-Robinson, D., Simms, I., Hay, P. 2010. "Randomised controlled trial of screening for Chlamydia trachomatis to prevent pelvic inflammatory disease: the POPI (prevention of pelvic infection) trial". *British medical journal*, 340:C1642.

[6] Baarda, B. I., Sikora, A. E. 2015. "Proteomics of Neisseria gonorrhoeae: the treasure hunt for countermeasures against an old disease". *Frontiers in microbiology,* 26; 6:1190.

[7] Ritter, J. L. 1., Genco, C. A2. 2018. "Neisseria gonorrhoeae–Induced Inflammatory Pyroptosis in Human Macrophages is Dependent on Intracellular Gonococci and Lipooligosaccharide". *Journal of cell death,* 3; 11:1179066017750902.

[8] Hebb, J. K. 1., Cohen, C. R., Astete, S. G., Bukusi, E. A., Totten, P. A. 2004. "Detection of novel organisms associated with salpingitis, by use of 16S rDNA polymerase chainreaction". *The Journal of infectious diseases,* 15; 190(12):2109 - 20.

[9] Baum, S., Sexton, D., Edwards, M. 2017. "*Mycoplasma hominis and Ureaplasma urealyticum infections*". URL: https://www.uptodate.com.

[10] Frobenius, W., Bogdan, C. 2015. "Diagnostic Value of Vaginal Discharge, Wet Mount and Vaginal pH – An Update on the Basics of Gynecologic Infectiology". *Geburtshilfe und Frauenheilkunde,* 75(4):355 - 366.

[11] Centers for Disease Control and Prevention. 2014. Recommendations for the laboratorybased detection of Chlamydia trachomatis and Neisseriagonorrhoeae -2014. *MMWR. Recommendations and reports: Morbidity and mortality weekly report. Recommendations and reports/Centers for Disease Control,* 14; 63(RR-02):1 - 19.

[12] Geisler, W. M. 2011. "Diagnosis and Management of Uncomplicated Chlamydia trachomatisInfections in Adolescents and Adults: Summary of Evidence Reviewed for the 2010 Centers for Disease Control and Prevention Sexually Transmitted Diseases Treatment Guidelines". *Clinical infectious diseases,* 53 Suppl. 3:S92-8.

[13] Cook, R. L., Hutchison, S. L., Østergaard, L., Braithwaite R. S., Ness RB. 2005. "Systematic review: noninvasive testing for

Chlamydia trachomatis and Neisseria gonorrhoeae". *Annals of internal medicine*, 7; 142(11):914 - 25.

[14] Greer, L., Wendel, G. D. Jr. 2008. "Rapid diagnostic methods in sexually transmitted infections". *Infectious disease clinics of North America,* 22(4):601 - 17.

[15] Low, N., Unemo, M., Skov Jensen, J., Breuer, J., Stephenson, J. M. 2014. "Molecular diagnostics for gonorrhoea: implications for antimicrobial resistance and the threat of untreatable gonorrhoea". *PLoS medicine*, 4; 11(2):e1001598.

[16] Whiley, D. M., Tapsall, J. W., Sloots, T. P. 2006. "Nucleic acid amplification testing for *Neisseria gonorrhoeae*: an ongoing challenge". *The Journal of molecular diagnostics.* 8(1): 3 - 15.

[17] Ona, S., Molina, R. L., Diouf, K. 2016. "Mycoplasma genitalium: An Overlooked Sexually Transmitted Pathogen in Women?". *Infectious diseases in obstetrics and gynecology*, 2016:4513089.

In: Pelvic Inflammatory Disease　　　　　ISBN: 978-1-53615-193-0
Editor: Daniel Abehsera　　　　　© 2019 Nova Science Publishers, Inc.

Chapter 4

RISK FACTORS:
ROUTES OF DISEASE TRANSMISSION

Marta de la Peña[*]*, MD, Marta Casaus, MD*
and Araceli Sánchez, MD
Obstetrics and Gynecology Department,
Quirónsalud Hospital, Málaga, Spain

Pelvic inflammatory disease (PID) is an infection of the female upper genital tract and describes a spectrum of infectious inflammatory disorders. It may involve any combination of the endometrium, fallopian tubes, ovaries, pelvic peritoneum and contiguous structures.

Any sexually active female is at risk for sexually transmitted infection (STI) associated pelvic inflammatory disease (PID), but those with multiple sexual partners are at the highest risk. Additionally, age younger than 25, a partner with a sexually transmitted infection, and a history of prior PID or a sexually transmitted infection are important risk factors. The use of barrier contraception is protective.

---

[*] Corresponding Author's Email: marta.dlp@quironsalud.es.

Table 1. Risk factors for pelvic inflammatory disease

Patient characteristics	Young patient age Low socioeconomic status Urban residence
Sexual behavior	Young age at first sexual intercourse Multiple sexual partners Concurrent sexual partners Number of new sexual partners in previous 30 days High frequency of sexual intercourse
Contraception	Barrier contraception Oral contraceptives IUD (intrauterine device) Tubal ligation
Prior and present infection	PID Gonorrhea Chlamydia Bacterial vaginosis
Vaginal douching	
Cigarette smoking	
Substances abuse	
Menstruation	

Source: self made.

African-American or Black-Caribbean ethnicity has been associated with a higher risk of PID. The reasons for this are likely multifactorial, possibly related to access to care or behavioral differences. These racial differences in PID risk may be decreasing over time.

In this chapter we will discuss many variables that have been identified that impact the risk of PID acquisition. A list of these risk factors is presented in Table 1.

1. PATIENT CHARACTERISTICS

Age is an independent risk factor for PID and is inversely related to the rate of PID. PID occurs in highest frequency among those 15 to 25 years of age; the incidence in women older than the age of 35 is only one-seventh that in younger women. Adolescents possess both biologic and behavioral characteristics that place them at greater risk for acquiring PID. Biologic factors include a lower prevalence of potentially protective chlamydial antibodies, a higher likelihood of anovulatory cycles with cervical mucus that is easier to penetrate, and larger zones of cervical ectopy with more columnar cells for which bacterial and viral infectious agents have a greater affinity. In terms of sexual behavior, sexually active teenagers are more likely than older women to have multiple and concurrent partners and may be more likely to have unprotected intercourse [1].

In Figure 1 are presented the rates of reported cases by age group of chlamydia and gonorrhea in the United States through 2016.

However, women aged 15 to 25 with PID appear to have less PID associated sequelae such as tubal damage and infertility than do older women with PID [2].

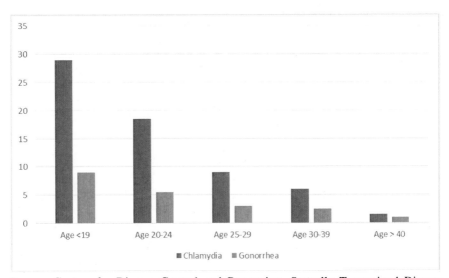

Source: Centers for Disease Control and Prevention. Sexually Transmitted Disease Surveillance 2016. Atlanta: U.S. Department of Health and Human Services; 2017.

Figure 1. Prevalence of Chlamydia and Gonorrhea by age group in the United States.

In addition to age, other demographic factors have been suggested as risk factors for developing PID. Socioeconomic measures such as low levels of education, unemployment, and low income have been associated with an increased risk. It has also been suggested that women who live in urban areas are at a higher risk for PID than those living in rural areas. Each of these risk factors may be markers for sexual behavior, and this is likely the basis for the association [1].

2. SEXUAL BEHAVIOR

Sex is the primary risk factor for PID. Celibate women are not at risk for PID, and women with longstanding monogamous relationships rarely develop PID. Sexual behaviors associated with increased PID risk include young age at first sexual intercourse, multiple sexual partners, number of new sexual partners in the previous 30 days and high frequency of sexual intercourse [1].

Young age at first sexual intercourse is associated with increased risk of PID, and may reflect biological factors and sexual behavior over a substantial period of time [3].

The number of sexual partners is one of the most important risk factors for the development of PID. Multiple sexual partners or a new partner may increase the risk of exposure to infectious agents. Some studies have confirmed multiple partners as a risk factor, associated with an increased frequency of PID ranging from 3 to 20 fold [4].

The frequency of intercourse has been associated with the development of PID in some studies. Increased frequency can increase exposure to both sexually transmitted pathogens and non-sexually transmitted organisms, such as group B *streptococci* [1].

3. CONTRACEPTION

Contraceptive choice has a large impact on the risk of developing sexually transmitted infections (STIs) and PID. Women who use no method of contraception are at an increased risk for STIs and PID, while consistent use of condoms offers a significant reduction of risk. Barrier contraception protects against PID. Condoms are the most effective form, preventing over 50 percent of endocervical gonococcal and chlamydial infections if used correctly. One large study suggested that consistent condom use following a diagnosis of PID could lower the rate of PID sequelae. Latex condoms provide greater protection than natural membrane condoms [1, 5].

Diaphragm use alone appears to decrease a woman's risk for PID, although it's precise protective effect against PID has not been determined because most women use spermicides with a diaphragm. The combination of spermicide and diaphragm, as well as other combinations of barrier methods, is expected to enhance protection against STIs and PID [2].

OCs have a complex interaction with PID. The association appears to be different for each link in the PID risk chain: increased risk of *Chlamydia trachomatis* and gonococcal infection of the endocervix, decreased risk of symptomatic PID, and no significant effect on risk of tubal infertility [2].

Several studies have shown that OC use nearly doubles the prevalence of both chlamydia and gonococcal infection of the cervix. The leading explanation for this observation is increased cervical ectropion induced by OCs (Figure 1). The greater area of columnar epithelium exposed on the vaginal aspect of the cervix may lead to a greater chance that infection will be acquired after sexual contact with an infected partner, and a greater number of susceptible columnar cells available for progressive growth cycles of the infective agent [6].

However, in the upper reproductive tract, OCs appear to provide some protection against symptomatic infection. The use of OCs has been shown to reduce the risk of PID by 40-60%. The mechanism for this protective effect remains speculative, but three explanations have been posited [7]:

- One is that thick cervical mucus, caused by the progestin component of combination OCs, provides a relatively impenetrable barrier to *Chlamydia trachomatis* and *Neisseria gonorrhoeae* in the lower genital tract.
- Another explanation is that decreased menstrual blood loss associated with OCs may produce a less than optimal environment for bacterial proliferation.
- Last, a recent explanation is that modifications of the immune responses to chlamydial infections or altered susceptibility of mucosal cells to *Chlamydia trachomatis* may be caused by OCs.

The concern that IUDs might causes or facilitate gynecologic infection has a long and controversial history [8]. The incidence rate of PID among IUD users depends heavily on the definition used and the means available for diagnosing PID. It varies from 1:100 to 1:1000 women per year [9].

There are some barriers prevent complete understanding of the role of the IUDs in a gynecologic infection [8, 9]:

- Asymptomatic infections: because an infection may produce mild or no symptoms, women may be inaccurately characterized as free of disease. This problem is particularly true for Chlamydia trachomatis, which can cause a significant number of asymptomatic cervical and upper genital tract infections.
- Timing of bacterial exposure in relation to insertion and use of an IUD: Presence of bacteria before the IUD is inserted can have

a completely different etiology compared to bacteria acquired after the IUD is in situ. Treatment of detected bacteria removes both the risk of infection.

- Imprecise diagnoses: It is difficult to obtain reliable information about whether use of IUDs is truly associated with increased risk of PID due to the complexity of diagnosis of PID correctly.
- Lack of appropriate comparison group: it is very difficult to identify a population or a control population in which the natural incidence of PID can be measured.

Event rates observed in natural history of PID may be altered by IUD use. The best evidence comes from a compilation of IUD studies conducted by the World Health Organization (WHO) [8, 9]. The data covered 22908 IUD insertions and 51,399 women-years of follow up. It was concluded that the incidence rate of PID in the first 20 days following the insertion of the IUD corresponded to 9.7/1000 women per year and the rate thereafter was flat 1.4/1000 women per year [8, 9]. These findings indicate that PID among IUD users is most strongly related to the insertion process and to background risk of sexually transmitted infection [10].

IUDs should be left in place up to their maximum lifespan and should not routinely be replaced earlier, provided that there are no contra-indications to continued use and the woman wishes to continue with the device [9].

Prophylactic antibiotics are generally not recommended for IUD insertion. This recommendation applies to healthy women The British Society for Antimicrobial Chemotherapy stated that antibiotic prophylaxis is not required for insertion or removal of IUD even in women with cardiac abnormalities or at risk of endocarditis [11].

Bacterial vaginosis has received much attention as being associated with the use of IUD and for being a possible precursor of PID. Several studies it has been reported that IUD users have higher rates of bacterial vaginosis when compared to women using other contraceptive method [8]. Recent study confirms that changes in the vaginal bacterial community composition were not associated with the use of Cu- IUD or LNG-IUS [10]. There isn´t a clear difference in vaginal microbiota stability with Cu- IUD versus LNG- IUS use [12].

Pelvic actinomycosis is a rare disease that can occur in women with a long duration of IUD use. Approximately 7% of women using an IUD may have a finding of actinomyces- like organisms on a Pap-test [24]. In the absence of symptoms, women with actinomyces-like organisms do no need antimicrobial treatment or IUD removal [13].

Women using the LNG-IUS had decrease numbers of CD4 cells expressing the HIV correceptor CCR5, in both endocervix and endometrium. [14]. Women use Cu IUD have similar results, suggesting that use of either type of IUD is associated with changes in T cells populations in the female genital tract that are not suggestive of an increased risk of HIV acquisition [14].

For women at high risk for HIV acquisition, HIV-infected women, HIV-infected IUCD users converting to an AIDS diagnosis and women with AIDS doing clinically well on highly active anti-retroviral therapy, both the copper and levonorgestrel-releasing system carry a WHO Level 2 recommendation. Dual-method condom use is still encouraged [9].

4. PRIOR OR PRESENT INFECTION

Secondary to ascension of lower genital tract organism into the uterus, fallopian tubes and peritoneal cavity, PID is most commonly caused by sexually transmitted pathogens, including *Chlamydia trachomatis* and *Neisseria gonorrhoeae* in 44 and 10% of cases, respectively. Dual infection is seen in approximately 12% of patients. The remaining cases are secondary to endogenous organisms including vaginal bacterial anaerobes and facultative bacteria [15].

The vaginal flora includes a variety of potentially pathogenic bacteria. Among these are species of *streptococcus, staphylococcus, Enterobacteriaceae* (most commonly *Klebsiella spp, Escherichia coli and Proteus spp*), and variety of anaerobes. Compared with the dominant *Lactobacillus spp,* these organism are present in low numbers, and ebb and flow under the influence of hormonal changes [16].

The endocervical canal functions as a barrier protecting the normally sterile upper genital tract from organism of the dynamic vaginal ecosystem. Endocervical infection with sexually transmitted pathogens can disrupt this barrier. The factor determining which cervical infections ascend to upper genital tract have not been completely elucidated, but data from prospective studies [17] suggest that about 15% of untreated chlamydial infections progress to clinically diagnosed pelvic inflammatory disease. The risk of PID after gonococcal infection may be even higher [17].

The mechanism by which gonorrhea and chlamydia cause damage to the fallopian tubes differs. In gonococcal PID there is a direct infection and destruction of the epithelial lining of the tube, with an acute inflammatory response usually leading to acute symptoms. Women with chlamydial disease have a more indolent clinical picture where much of the tubal damage occurs secondary to immune response to infection, as result of cross reactivity between human and chlamydia proteins [18].

Women with pelvic infection often also have a bacterial vaginosis. In bacterial vaginosis there is an imbalance in the vaginal flora with loss of lactobacilli and increase in other bacterial species, including *Gardnerella, Mobiluncus* and anaerobes, associated with an offensive vaginal discharge [19]. Bacterial vaginosis is associated with local production of enzymes that degrade the cervical mucus and associated antimicrobial peptides. This degradation may impair the cervical barrier to ascending infection and facilitate the spread of microorganisms to the upper genital tract [19]. Women presenting initially with bacterial vaginosis do not appear to be at an increased risk of developing PID, with two exceptions [16]:

- First, those who have large quantities of Gram negative anaerobes in the vaginal have a slightly increased risk of developing upper genital infection.
- Second, those with bacterial vaginosis who subsequently acquire gonorrhea or chlamydia are also increased risk.

5. VAGINAL DOUCHING

The importance of a healthy vaginal micro-flora is indisputable. Therefore, intravaginal practices, such as vaginal douching, may inhibit or lower the colonization of beneficial Lactobacilli strains.

Douching has been linked to gonococcal or chlamydial cervicitis and PID in retrospective studies. The authors [20] conducted a 1999-2004 prospective observational study of 1,199 US women who were at high risk of acquiring *chlamydia* and were followed for up to 4 years. Cervical *Neisseria gonorrhoeae* and *Chlamydia trachomatis* were detected from vaginal swabs by nucleic acid amplification. PID was characterized by histologic endometritis or pelvic pain and tenderness plus one of the following: oral temperature >38.3 degrees C, leucorrhea or mucopus, erythrocyte sedimentation rate >15 mm/hour, white blood cell count >10,000, or gonococcal/chlamydial lower genital tract infection. Associations between douching and PID or gonococcal/chlamydial genital infections were assessed by proportional hazards models. The 4-year incidence rate of PID was 10.9% and of gonococcal and/or chlamydial cervicitis was 21.9%. After adjustment for confounding factors, douching two or more times per month at baseline was associated with neither PID (adjusted hazard ratio = 0.76, 95% confidence interval: 0.42, 1.38) nor gonococcal/chlamydial genital infection (adjusted hazard ratio = 1.16, 95% confidence interval: 0.76, 1.78). Frequency of douching immediately preceding PID or gonococcal/chlamydial genital infection was not different between women who developed versus did not develop outcomes. These data do not support an association between douching and development of PID or gonococcal/chlamydial genital infection among predominantly young, African-American women.

6. CIGARETTE SMOKING

Cigarette smoking has been implicated as a risk factor for PID sequelae, but the association between smoking and PID has yet to be fully examined. A study conducted a population-based case-control to evaluate smoking as a risk factor for acute PID [21]. The case patients (n = 131) were women Health Maintenance Organization (HMO) enrollees between the ages of 18 and 40 years who were treated for a first episode of PID. The control patients (n = 294) were randomly selected from the HMO enrollment files. Relative to never smokers, current smokers were at increased risk of PID. Women who smoked 10 or more cigarettes per day had a higher risk than did those who smoked less. Available data indicate that smoking status is not serving as a marker for uncontrolled confounding by lifestyle factors. These study results suggest that smoking represents a modifiable risk factor for acute PID.

7. SUBSTANCES ABUSE

Multiples studies have demonstrated the strong correlation between substance abuse and sexual behaviors that put individuals at risk for STIs [22, 23]. A study about substance abuse treatment facility in Alabama, 40% of women and 15% of men reported having ever exchanged sex for drugs, while 53% of women and 36% of men reported a history of STIs [24]. Despite the documented high STI risk for substance abusers, few studies have examined the prevalence of STIs among individuals seeking substance abuse treatment. Such studies may not have been conducted in the past due to a general lack of emphasis on medical issues in substance abuse treatment and because traditional methods of STI testing have been unwieldy, requiring penile urethral swabs or pelvic examinations. In addition, STI screening may be challenging to accomplish in patient substance abuse detoxification programs as typical length of stay is brief, 4–6 days. Despite the appeal of using non-invasive methods to screen all clients for STIs in substance abuse treatment programs, the unexpectedly low prevalence of *C. trachomatis* and *N. gonorrhoeae* in this study suggests that widespread screening is not indicated. In other locales, higher STI prevalence in the general population may persuade public health officials to consider screens for STIs in substance abuse treatment programs, particularly in detoxification programs [24].

8. MENSTRUATION

PID is a common and serious complication of sexually transmitted diseases in young women but is rarely diagnosed in the postmenopausal woman. The epidemiology of PID, as well as the changes that occur in the genital tract of postmenopausal women, explain this discrepancy. The exact incidence of PID in postmenopausal women is unknown; however, in one series, fewer than 2% of women with tuboovarian abscess formation were postmenopausal [25]. With menopause, the cervical transformation zone is anatomically located within the endocervical canal and is smaller than in premenopausal women, decreasing the area of attachment available to *C. trachomatis and N. gonorrhoeae*. These changes most likely lower the susceptibility of the postmenopausal woman to infection. The endocervix also acts as a functional barrier to ascending infection. This barrier can be attenuated by the changing rheological properties of the cervical mucus as noted during ovulation or breached by the occurrence of retrograde menstruation. Physiologically, the cervical mucus of the menopausal woman is more tenacious and serves as a mechanical barrier to ascending infections. Lack of menstruation in menopausal women decreases the risk of infection of the upper genital tract.

9. PID BY CONTIGUITY

The direct extension of infectious processes from adjacent intraabdominal viscera is more likely to be associated with PID in older women. Disorders such as diverticulitis, Crohn disease, colonic cancers, and appendicitis have been associated with a direct spread of infection to the ovaries, oviducts, and uterus and manifest as a unilateral or bilateral tuboovarian abscess. Fistula formation from an abscess cavity to the genital tract has also been described [25].

REFERENCES

[1] Zenilman J, Shahmanesh M. 2012. *"Sexually transmitted infections."* Sudbury, Mass: Jones & Bartlett Learning.
[2] Washington A. 1991. "Assessing Risk for Pelvic Inflammatory Disease and Its Sequelae." *JAMA: The Journal of the American Medical Association*; 266(18),2581.
[3] Simms I, Stephenson JM, Mallinson H, Peeling RW, Thomas K, Gokhale R, Rogers PA, Hay P, Oakeshott P, Hopwood J, Birley H, Hernon M. 2006. "Risk factors associated with pelvic inflammatory disease." *Sexually transmitted infections*, 82(6),452-457.
[4] Kreisel K, Torrone E, Bernstein K, Hong J, Gorwitz R. 2017. "Prevalence of Pelvic Inflammatory Disease in Sexually Experienced Women of Reproductive Age — United States, 2013–2014." *CDC MMWR Morbidity and Mortality Weekly Report*; 66(3),80-83.

[5]   Ness R, Randall H, Richter H, Peipert J, Montagno A, Soper D, Sweet R, Nelson D, Schubeck D, Hendrix S, Bass D, Kip K. 2004. "Condom Use and the Risk of Recurrent Pelvic Inflammatory Disease, Chronic Pelvic Pain, or Infertility Following an Episode of Pelvic Inflammatory Disease." *American Journal of Public Health*, 94(8), 1327-1329.

[6]   Louv W, Austin H, Perlman J, Alexander W. 1989. "Oral contraceptive use and the risk of chlamydial and gonococcal infections." *American Journal of Obstetrics and Gynecology*, 160(2),396-402.

[7]   Wolner-Hanssen P. 1990. "Decreased risk of symptomatic chlamydial pelvic inflammatory disease associated with oral contraceptive use." *JAMA: The Journal of the American Medical Association*, 263(1),54-59.

[8]   Hubacher D. 2014. "Intrauterine devices & infection: Review of literature." *The Indian journal of medical research*; 140(Suppl1): S53-S57.

[9]   Martinez F, López-Arregui E. 2009. "Infection risk and intrauterine devices." *Acta Obstetricia et Gynecologica Scandinavica*; 88:246-250.

[10] Farley TM, Rosenberg MJ, Rowe PJ, Chen JH, Meirik O. 1992. "Intrauterine devices and pelvic inflammatory disease: an international perspective." *Lancet*; 339:785-788.

[11] National Institute for Health and Clinical Excellence. 2008. "*NICE Clinical Guideline 64: prophylaxis against infective endocarditis*." URL: https://www.nice.org.uk/guidance/cg64.

[12] Bassis CM, Allsworth JE, Wahl HN, Sack DE, Young VB, Bell JD. 2017. "Effects of intrauterine contraception on the vaginal microbiota." *Contraception*; 96(3):189-195.

[13] Nakahira ES, Maximiano LF, Lima FR. 2017. "Abdominal and pelvic actinomycosis due to longstanding intrauterine device: a slow and devastating infection." *Autopsy and Case Reports*; 7(1):43-47.

[14] Achilles SL, Creinin MD, Stoner KA, Chen BA, Meyn L, Hillier SL. 2014. "Changes in genital tract inmune cell population after initiation of intrauterine contraception." *American Journal of Obstetrics & Gynecology*; 211(5):489.e1-489.e9.

[15] Spain J, Rheinboldt M. 2017. "MDCT of pelvic inflammatory disease: a review of the pathophysiology, gamut of imaging findings, and treatment." *Emergency Radiology;* 24, 87-93.

[16] Haggerty CL, Hillier SL, Bass DC, Ness RB. 2004. "Bacterial vaginosis and anaerobic bacteria are associated with endometritis." *Clinical infectius disease*; 39,990-95.

[17] Robert C, Bruham MD, Sami L, Gottilieb MD. 2015. "Pelvic inflammatory Disease." *The New England Journal of Medicine*; 372, 2039-2048.

[18] Price MJ, Ades AE, De Angelis D, Welton NJ, Macleod J, Soldan K, Simms I, Turner K, Horner PJ. 2013. "Risk of pelvic inflammatory disease following Clamydia trachomatis infection: analysis of prospective studies with a multistate model." *American Journal of Epidemiology*; 178,484-492.

[19] Ness RB, Kip KE, Hillier SL, Soper DE, Stamm CA, Sweet RL, Rice P, Richter HE. 2005. "A cluster analysis of bacterial vaginosis associated microflora and pelvic inflammatory disease." *American Journal of Epidemiology*; 166, 585-590.

[20] Simpson T, Merchant J, Grimley DM, Oh MK. 2004. "Vaginal douching among adolescent and young women: more challenges than progress." *Journal of pediatric and adolescent gynecology*; 17(4):249-55.

[21] Scholes D, Daling J, Stergachis A. 1992. "Current cigarette smoking and risk of acute pelvic inflammatory disease." *American journal of public health*; 82(10)1352–1355.

[22] Bagnall G, Plant M, Warwick W. 1990. "Alcohol, drugs and AIDS-related risks: results from a prospective study." *AIDS Care*; 2(4)309–317.

[23] Poulin C, Alary M, Bernier F, Ringuet J, Joly J. 1999. "Prevalence of *Chlamydia trachomatis*, *Neisseria gonorrhoeae*, and HIV infection among drug users attending an STD/HIV prevention and needle-exchange program in Quebec City, Canada." *Sexually transmitted diseases*; 26(7)410–420.

[24] Bachmann L, Lewis I, Allen R, Schwebke JR, Leviton LC, Siegal HA, Hooke EW 3rd. 2000. "Risk and prevalence of treatable sexually transmitted disease at a Birmingham substance abuse treatment facility." *American journal of public health;* 90(10):1615–1618.

[25] Brunham RC, Gottlieb SL, Paavonen J. 2015. "Pelvic Inflammatory Disease." *The New England journal of medicine;* 372(21):2039-48.

In: Pelvic Inflammatory Disease   ISBN: 978-1-53615-193-0
Editor: Daniel Abehsera   © 2019 Nova Science Publishers, Inc.

Chapter 5

COMPLEMENTARY TESTS IN PELVIC INFLAMMATORY DISEASE

Raquel P. Duarte*, MD, PhD, Aurelia Marsac, MD and Lourdes Martínez, MD
Obstetrics and Gynecology Department,
Quirónsalud Hospital, Málaga, Spain

1. INTRODUCTION

The pelvic inflammatory disease (PID) represents a spectrum of infection and there is no single diagnostic gold standard. PID should be suspected in any young or sexually active female patient who presents with pelvic discomfort. The absence of findings in complementary tests does not necessarily roll out PID.

Because PID is a clinical diagnosis, laboratory tests or imaging studies are not usually necessary, but they can be helpful in establishing

---

* Corresponding Author's Email: raquelp.duarte@quironsalud.es.

the diagnosis, defining its severity, or in monitor the response to treatment [1].

2. LABORATORY TESTS

The following tests should be performed for all women suspected of PID:

- Pregnancy test.
- Microscopy of vaginal discharge.
- Nucleic acid amplification tests (NAATs) for *Chlamydia trachomatis, Neisseria gonorrhoeae,* and *Mycoplasma genitalium.*
- Sexual transmission diseases screening including HIV and syphilis.

Most laboratory findings in PID are nonspecific. The first test that should be done is a pregnancy test. It is very important to differentiate between PID and a possible ectopic pregnancy or, less common, a complication of an intrauterine pregnancy.

It should also be performed a microscopic examination of vaginal discharge and NAATs for *Chlamydia trachomatis, Neisseria gonorrhoeae* and *Mycoplasma genitalium,* since a positive result supports the diagnosis of PID. However, its absence from the endocervix or urethra does not exclude PID [2, 3].

Mycoplasma genitalium is a sexually transmitted pathogen that is emerging among women diagnosed with PID. In some populations studied, infection with *Mycoplasma genitalium* is as common as *Chlamydia trachomatis* among high risk sexually active women. Although PID has a polymicrobial etiology, with *Chlamydia trachomatis* and/or *Neisseria gonorrhoeae* isolated from approximately one-third to one half of cases [4, 5], many PID cases have an unidentified etiology. The symptoms characteristic of nongonococcal, nonchlamydial PID have not been well described. In a study of women with clinically suspected PID, women with *Mycoplasma genitalium* infection were less likely to have elevated systemic inflammatory markers and fever in comparison with gonococcal PID. Also, those women were less likely to present with mucopurulent cervicitis and high pelvic pain score. However, women with chlamydial PID had signs and symptoms that were similar to those in women with M. genitalium infection [6]. The microbiologic diagnosis of *Mycoplasma genitalium* infection is infrequent because of the lack of approved standard test; most are done with PCR detection since the culture of the pathogen is very fastidious. It is mostly important to adapt antibiotic therapy. This pathogen is naturally resistant to penicillin and other betalactams but generally sensible to macrolides, fluoroquinolones, tetracyclines and clindamycin, even though resistance is a growing issue [7].

Saline microscopy of vaginal discharge or vaginal smear is to assess for increased white blood cells in vaginal fluid, which is sensitive for PID [8]. In a cohort of women at high risk for pelvic infections, absence of vaginal white blood cells had excellent negative predictive value (95%) [9]. These data suggest that if an evaluation of a saline microscopy of vaginal fluid reveals no white blood cells (leucorrhea), an alternative diagnosis to PID should be considered. On the other hand, the presence of white blood cells in vaginal fluid has a poor positive predictive value, around 17% [9] so their presence is not specific to PID.

A complete blood count, erythrocyte sedimentation rate (ESR), and C-reactive protein (CRP) are often obtained in patients with middle to severe clinical presentation including fever and who may need inpatient treatment [3]. In the PEACH trial, which enrolled women with abdominal pain, pelvic tenderness and evidence of lower genital tract inflammation, an elevated leukocyte count ($\geq$ 10,000 cells/mL) had 41% sensitivity and 76% specificity for the presence of endometritis [8]. In another cohort study, an elevated erythrocyte sedimentation rate (>

15mm/h) had 70% sensitivity and 52% specificity for endometritis or salpingitis [9]. PID is usually an acute process, only a minority of PID patients with more severe disease exhibit peripheral blood leukocytosis [11]. PID diagnosis is supported by an increase of white blood cell, CRP or ESR, but these parameters could be normal; they can be used to assess severity and monitor the response to treatment. In a study of 38 women with severe case of PID, it had been observed a negative correlation between the leukocyte count at admission and the need for surgical treatment. [12] This could be explained by the fact that those cases may be were more sub-acute or chronic and so the antibiotic therapy was not as effective as it is in acute cases of PID.

It is also highly recommended to *screen for other sexually transmitted diseases* such as syphilis, hepatitis B and C, or HIV. HIV-infected women are associated with higher risk of tubo-ovarian abscess [13].

Recommend removal of an intrauterine device (IUD) present at the time of diagnosis of acute PID is controversial. A single randomized controlled trail suggests that it may improve the rate of successful treatment. In contrast other authors, in a subsequent systematic review, find little difference in outcomes for women with mild to-moderate PID who retain their IUD in situ during treatment. These studies primarily included women using copper or other nonhormonal IUDs. No studies are available regarding treatment outcomes in women using levonorgestrel-releasing IUDs. If no clinical improvement occurs within 48–72 hours of initiating treatment, providers should consider removing the IUD. [3] Most studies seem to agree that there is insufficient evidence to recommend empiric removal. Caution should be exercise if the IUD stays in place and close monitoring is required.

Current partners of women with PID should be screened for *Neisseria gonorrhoeae, Chlamydia trachomatis* (and *Mycoplasma genitalium* if the index patient is infected). If screening is positive in the male partner, treatment should be administered appropriately and concurrently with the index patient. Because many cases of PID are not associated with *Neisseria gonorrhoeae, Chlamydia trachomatis* or *Mycoplasma genitalium*, broad spectrum empirical therapy should also be offered to male partners (Doxycycline 100 mg twice daily for one week) and should be advised to avoid unprotected intercourse until they and their partner have completed the treatment course [10].

3. IMAGING TECHNIQUES

3.1. Ultrasound

Ultrasound is a low cost complementary test, and has no negative effects or exposure to radiation, but also produces high quality images of the upper genital tract in its transvaginal modality; these are some of the reasons why it is widely used to help diagnose PID, even as a first election imaging technique. In the early phase of infection, it is common for ultrasound appearances to be normal. As the disease advances, ultrasound can demonstrate uterine enlargement and thickening of the endometrium. It can also show the loss of tissue plains and an ill-defined uterus [14].

The interpretation of sonographic findings is operator-dependent. Some authors tried to identify the most commonly observed and reproducible ones [15-17]. For example, a thickened fluid-filled tube with or without free pelvic fluid, had a sensitivity of 85% and a specificity of 100% for endometritis among women with clinically diagnosed PID [15]. Timor-Tritsch identified acute tubal inflammatory disease by the following transvaginal sonographic markers: Shape, wall structure (incomplete septa, "cogwheel" sign or the "beads-on- a-string" sign), wall thickness (≥5mm) and presence of pelvic peritoneal fluid, like free fluid or inclusion cyst. The best marker of tubal inflammatory disease, either acute or chronic, was the presence of an incomplete septum of the tubal wall, which was present in 92% of the total cases [16]. Incomplete septum is defined as hyperechoic septa that originate as a triangular protrusion from one of the wall, but do not reach the opposite wall.

Romosan tried to sum up current knowledge on the sensitivity and specificity of ultrasound features suggestive of acute pelvic inflammatory disease. Upon reviewing seven articles, the presence of "thick tubal walls" proved to be a specific and sensitive ultrasound sign of acute PID, but only if the walls of the tubes could be evaluated. [17] Thickened longitudinal folds produce a characteristic "cogwheel" appearance when imaged in cross section. These folds can be mistaken for mural nodules on transverse images of the fallopian tube [18]. The "cogwheel" sign is also a specific sign of PID (95–99% specificity), but it seems to be less sensitive (0–86% sensitivity).

Hydrosalpinx or pyosalpinx is a common complication of salpingitis. Ultrasound can identify dilated fallopian tubes containing heterogenous fluid with echogenic debris; features typical of pyosalpinx. The fallopian tubes may be folded and demonstrate areas of tube tapering, and intraluminal small linear echogenic foci may be visualized. As pyosalpinx develops into tubo-ovarian abscesses, echogenic debris can be seen in the fallopian tubes and ovaries, representing inflammatory exudates, blood and pus [14].

Doppler results overlap too much between women with and without acute PID for them to be useful in the diagnosis of acute PID, even though acutely inflamed tubes are richly vascularized at color Doppler.

Additional imaging studies will be used in case of atypical symptoms, the patient does not improve after 72 hours of empiric antibiotic treatment, or when there is persistent pain after completing treatment. These findings suggest a complication of PID such as un tubo-ovarian abscess or an alternate diagnostic.

Table 1. General recommendations

PID diagnostic is mostly clinical.
Pregnancy test
Hemogram with erythrocyte sedimentation rate and C-reactive protein
Screening for other sexually transmitted infection (HIV and syphilis)
Vaginal smear
Endocervical swab (at least 3 samples: mycoplasma and chlamydia detection and bacterial culture)
Remove intrauterine device if no clinical improvement after 3 days of treatment
Partner screening and treatment

Table 2. Imaging techniques comparation

Ultrasound	Computariced tomography	Magnetic resonance
Cheap	Available	Not widely available
Available	Disadvantage: radiation	Confussing adnexal mass or
Prior test	Differential diagnosis	chronical episodes

3.2. Computerized Tomography

PID symptoms are frequently unspecific and may lead to differential diagnosis. At the emergency service contest of an incoming woman with low abdominal pain, the first image test that should be done is ultrasound, but in many cases, even though it is not the prior option, these patients will undergo a computerized tomography (CT) to assess the origin of the pathology (after a negative pregnancy test in fertile age women). CT will help us to determine the illness extension, identify associated complications, evaluate patients non-responding to antibiotics or to decide if it is possible a percutaneous drainage ultrasound or CT guided. [18-20].

CT findings in acute PID are [18-21]:

- Initial PID
  - Normal TC
  - Pelvic inflammatory changes: uterosacral ligaments thickening, pelvic oedema with erasing of the fat line; and highlight of periovarian peritoneum.
  - Salpingitis. Fallopian tubes show a thickening of the wall and may be filled. Most specific CT finding for acute PID is thickening of both fallopian tubes instead of unilateral one [22].
  - Ooforitis. Enhancement of ovarian and they may look polycystic.
  - Endometritis: abnormal endometrial enhancement and simple fluid.
  - Cervicitis, with enhancement of the channel walls.
  - Liquid in pouch of Douglas.
- Advanced PID:
  - Pyosalpinx/Hydrosalpinx: tubular juxtauterine mass filled with complex fluid (pus), with thickening and enhancing of tube walls. (Figure 15). Hydrosalpinx may be due also to chronic PID and may be seen incidentally at CT. Tubal and peritubal adhesions with fimbria obstruction produces the image called" beak sign."
  - Tube-ovarian abscess: thickened wall collections liquid filled, with septums, liquid levels, detritus and although internal gas finding is uncommon, it is relatively specific for tube-ovarian abscess (Figure 1).
- Contiguous structures affection:
  - Dilation of small or large bowel, producing ileus and even obstruction because of inflammation, oedema and attachment of pelvic structures.

- Ureteral obstruction.

- Gonadal vein thrombosis.

- Fitz-Hugh-Curtis syndrome. Inflammation of right hypochondrium and right hepatic lobe, with enhancement of hepatic capsule. Inflammation of the Glisson capsule can cause subcapsular and periportal geographic areas of perfusional variation. Gallbladder wall thickening may be present. There may be peritoneal septa and loculated perihepatic fluid such as adherences in abdominal wall and hepatic surface seen in surgery as "violin cords."

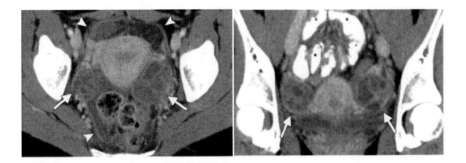

Figure 1. Contrast enhanced CT show bilateral complex cystic masses (arrows) with thick enhancing walls and septa, along with inflammation of the pelvic fat and peritoneum (arrowheads).

Appendicitis is one of the most frequent differential diagnosis for PID. In CT imaging, images associated to PID such as tubal thickening and pelvic fat haziness can be found also in appendicitis. One of the most common differential diagnosis in these women is appendicitis vs PID. There is a recent study [23] that states two main radiological CT signs to differentiate PID from appendicitis. This study has concluded that only two CT findings in all the studied are accurate to differentiate PID from appendicitis: appendiceal diameter >7mm and thickening of left tube. According to their decision tree, when there is inflammatory acute pain in women, the appendix must be evaluated in the CT on the beginning; if the appendiceal diameter is <7mm, appendicitis is improbable so PID findings should be investigated (tubal thickening -specially left tube-, anterior pelvic fat stranding, uterine serosal enhancement, inner myometrial enhancement, obliteration of presacral and perirectal fascial planes, loss of definition of the uterine border and pelvic peritoneal enhancement).

3.3. Magnetic Resonance Imaging

Magnetic Resonance (MR) is an image test not widely available, especially in emergency services, so its use in acute PID is limited. The power of MR in adnexal pathology is its capacity to identify the ovary, demonstrate tubular nature of a structure, and differentiate pyosalpinx from hemathosalpinx [18]. Even though some authors try to demonstrate that MR is comparable to laparoscopy and superior to clinical evaluation or ultrasound in PID diagnosis [24], present evidence is that CT or MR are not better than ultrasound in acute PID, but they are worthy in subacute or atypical pathogen cases, such us tuberculosis, actinomices, etc. [25]. MR findings of PID are tubo-ovarian abscesses, pyosalpinx, liquid inside the tubes or free liquid in pelvis [26].

In moderate acute PID the MR will show pyosalpinx or tubo-ovarian abscesses. When there is pyosalpinx, the image shows liquid-particles levels and highlighting of the wall after intravenous contrast, with a thickened and inflamed wall that shows hypointense or heterogeneous image in T1 (depending on the protein content of the fluid) sequences and hyperintense in T2 [18]. The tube-ovarian abscess (Figure 2) is a rounded/tubular liquid lesion with thick walls, T1 hyperintense thin internal line with hypointense content (if there is haemorrhagic material can be hyperintense), T2 hypointense with septa and intense post-gadolinium absorption [18, 20, 27].

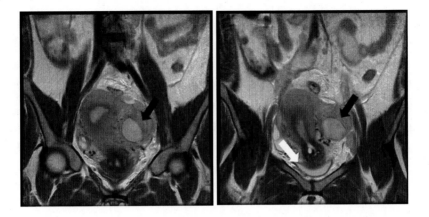

Figure 2. Tubo-ovarian abscesses. Left: tubo-ovarian abscess (black arrow). Right: Tubo-ovarian abscess (black arrow) and Douglas pouch abscess (white arrow).

Chronic PID usually shows like an adnexal mass due to hydrosalpinx; the use of MR is the key to differentiate this entity from peritoneal inclusion cyst [18]. Hydrosalpinx image is a "S" or "C" shaped tortuous tube structures that show liquid signal in T1 (hypointense) and T2 (hyperintense) sequences, with specific thin mucous longitudinal folding [18, 27]; the wall can be thickened or thin, no absorption of the contrast in the wall and no contiguous inflammation [20].

4. OTHER TESTS

Findings on laparoscopy or transcervical endometrial biopsy can confirm the clinical diagnosis of PID [11], but these tests are uncommonly performed because of their invasiveness.

4.1. Laparoscopy

Laparoscopy is sometimes indicated in the evaluation of acute pelvic pain, especially when the diagnosis is not clear after less invasive evaluations; then, laparoscopy is useful to confirm the diagnosis of PID but also to identify the pathogen, because samples are not contaminated as could happen in vaginal samples [26]. Most women with acute pelvic pain, normal imaging and laboratory studies, and a normal physical examination will improve without need for intervention. Gynecological diagnoses that may be missed in these patients include subclinical pelvic inflammatory disease [28-29]. According to laparoscopy findings, PID can be classified in different grades [26]:

- I: erythema in tubal serosa
- II: peritoneal liquid or evidence of purulent secretion by the tubes
- III: tubo-ovarian abscese
- IV: breaking of the tuboovarian abscese

Despite its value in confirming a diagnosis of PID, laparoscopy is not sensitive enough to be considered the diagnostic gold standard. The specificity of laparoscopy is high, but its sensitivity is as low as 50 percent when compared with fimbrial histopathology because it does not detect isolated endometritis or mild intra-tubal inflammation [30]. Additionally, it is an invasive procedure, particularly for a condition that does not typically warrant surgical intervention.

4.2. Transcervical Endometrial Biopsy

Histologic evidence of endometritis on transcervical endometrial biopsy can help to confirm the diagnosis and may in fact detect early cases not yet visible at laparoscopy [31]. However, it is not used routinely because the correlation between endometritis and salpingitis is not 100 percent [11].

Endometrial biopsy findings usually confirm the presence of infection but rarely identify the causative organism. Chronic endometritis is more commonly seen than acute endometritis [32].

REFERENCES

[1] Kahn JG, Walker CK, Washington AE, Landers DV, Sweet RL. 1991. "Diagnosing pelvic inflammatory disease. A comprehensive analysis and considerations for developing a new model." *Journal of American Medical Association (JAMA)*; 266(18):2594–604.

[2] Bevan CD, Johal BJ, Mumtaz G, Ridgway GL, Siddle NC. 1995. "Clinical, laparoscopic and microbiological findings in acute salpingitis: report on a United Kingdom cohort." *British Journal of Obstetrics & Gynaecology*; 102(5):407-414.

[3] Workowski KA, Bolan GA. 2015. "Centers for Disease Control and Prevention. Sexually transmitted diseases treatment guidelines." *Morbidity and Mortality Weekly Report. Recommendations and reports (MMWR Recomm Rep)*; 64:1.

[4] Simms I, Eastick K, Mallinson H, Thomas K, Gokhale R, Hay P, Herring A, Rogers PA. 2003. "Associations between Mycoplasma genitalium, Chlamydia trachomatis and pelvic inflammatory disease." *Journal of Clinical Pathology*; 56(8):616–618.

[5] Ness RB, Soper DE, Holley RL, Peipert J, Randall H, Sweet RL, Sondheimer SJ, Hendrix SL, Amortegui A, Trucco G, Songer T, Lave JR, Hillier SL, Bass DC, Kelsey SF. 2002. "Effectiveness of inpatient and outpatient treatment strategies for women with pelvic inflammatory disease: results from the Pelvic Inflammatory Disease Evaluation and Clinical Health (PEACH) randomized trial." *American Journal of Obstetrics and Gynecology*; 186(5):929–937.

[6]   Short VL, Totten PA, Ness RB, Astete SG, Kelsey SF, Haggerty CL. 2009. "Clinical presentation of Mycoplasma genitalium Infection versus Neisseria gonorrhoeae infection among women with pelvic inflammatory disease." *Clinical infectious diseases*; 48:41.

[7]   Taylor-Robinson D, Jensen JS. 2011. "Mycoplasma genitalium: from Chrysalis to multicolored butterfly." *Clinical microbiology reviews*; 24(3):498-514.

[8]   Peipert JF, Ness RB, Blume J, Soper DE, Holley R, Randall H, Sweet RL, Sondheimer SJ, Hendrix SL, Amortegui A, Trucco G, Bass DC; Pelvic Inflammatory Disease Evaluation and Clinical Health Study Investigators. 2001. "Clinical predictors of endometritis in women with symptoms and signs of pelvic inflammatory disease." *American Journal of Obstetrics and Gynecology*; 184(5):856–63. discussion 63-4.

[9]   Yudin MH, Hillier SL, Wiesenfeld HC, Krohn MA, Amortegui AA, Sweet RL. 2003. "Vaginal polymorphonuclear leukocytes and bacterial vaginosis as markers for histologic endometritis among women without symptoms of pelvic inflammatory disease." *American Journal of Obstetrics and Gynecology*; 188(2):318–23.

[10] Ross J, Guaschino S, Cusini M, Jensen J. 2018. "2017 European guideline for the management of pelvic inflammatory disease." *International journal of STD & AIDS*; 29:108.

[11] Ross J, Chacko MR. 2018. "Pelvic inflammatory disease: Clinical manifestations and diagnosis." *Up to date*. URL: https://www.uptodate.com/contents/pelvic-inflammatory-disease-clinical-manifestations-and-diagnosis.

[12] Abehsera D, Panal M, Sánchez M, Herrera M, de Santiago FJ. 2013. "Outcome after action protocol in severe pelvic inflammatory disease patients." *Ginecología y obstetricia de México*; 81(6):304-309.

[13] Cohen CR, Sinei S, Reilly M, Bukusi E, Eschenbach D, Holmes KK, Ndinya-Achola JO, Bwayo J, Grieco V, Stamm W, Karanja J,

Kreiss J. 1998. "Effect of human immunodeficiency virus type 1 infection upon acute salpingitis: A laparoscopic study." *The Journal of Infectious Diseases*; 178(5):1352–8.

[14] Roche O, Chavan N, Aquilina J. Rockall A. 2012. "Radiological appearances of gynaecological emergencies." *Insights Imaging*; 3(3):265-75.

[15] Cacciatore B, Leminen A, Ingman-Friberg S, Ylostalo P, Paavonen J. 1992. "Transvaginal sonographic findings in ambulatory patients with suspected pelvic inflammatory disease." *Obstetrics and Gynecology*; 80(6):912–6.

[16] Timor-Tritsch IE, Lerner JP, Monteagudo A, Murphy KE, Heller DS. 1998. "Transvaginal sonographic markers of tubal inflammatory disease." *Ultrasound in Obstetrics and Gynecology*; 12(1):56–66.

[17] Romosan G, Valentin L. 2014. "The sensitivity and specificity of transvaginal ultrasound with regard to acute pelvic inflammatory disease: a review of the literature." *Archives of Gynecology and Obstetrics*; 289:705.

[18] Rezvani M, Shaaban AM. 2011. "Fallopian tube disease in the nonpregnant patient." *Radiograhics*; 31:527-548.

[19] Alcalde Odriozola, Castillo de Juan, Nates Uribe, Viteri Jusué, Schuller Arteaga, Grande Icaran. 2014. "Usefulness of CT in pelvic inflammatory disease." Poster presented in the *biannual meeting of Sociedad Española Radiología Médica*. Bilbao, Spain, May 22-25. DOI: 10.1594/seram2014/S-1058.

[20] Rojas Jiménez, Otero García, Trillo Fandiño, Caldera Díaz, Blanco Lobato. 2012. "Pelvic inflammatory disease pathways and their radiologycal find spectrum" Poster presented in the *biannual meeting of Sociedad Española Radiología Médica*. Granada, Spain, May 25-28. DOI: 10.1594/seram2012/S-0422.

[21] Sam JW, Jacobs JE, Birnbaum BA. 2002." Spectrum of CT Findings in Acute Pyogenic Pelvic Inflammatory Disease." *RadioGraphics*; 22:1327–1334.

[22] Jung SI, Kim YJ, Park HS, Jeon HJ, Jeong KA. "Acute pelvic inflammatory disease: Diagnostic performance of CT." 2010. *Journal of Obstetriscs and Gynaecology Research*; (37)3:228–235.

[23] El Hentour K, Millet I, Pages-Bouic E, Curros-Doyon F, Molinari N, Taourel P. 2018. "How to differentiate acute pelvic inflammatory disease from acute appendicitis? A decision tree based on CT findings." *European Radiology*; 28:673–682.

[24] Tukeva TA, Aronen HJ, Karjalainen PT, Molander P, Paavonen T, Paavonen J. 1999. MR imaging in pelvic inflammatory disease: comparison with laparoscopy and US. *Radiology*; 210(1):209-16.

[25] Huete A, Craig J, Vial C, Farías M, Tsunekawa H, Cuello M. 2016. "Imaging role in benign gynecological pathology process." *Revista Chilena de Obstetricia y Ginecología*; 81(1): 63 – 85.

[26] Saona-Ugarte P. 2007. "Pelvic inflammatory disease: diagnosis and complications." *Revista Peruana de Ginecología y Obstetricia*; 53:234-239.

[27] Llaverías Borrell S, Gallart Ortuño A, Querol Borrás V, Mundt E, Mauri Paytubi E, Maristany Daunert MT. 2014. "Magnetic Resonance in adnexal benign mass characterization: image find and differential diagnosis." Poster presented in *the biannual meeting of Sociedad Española Radiología Médica*. Bilbao, Spain, May 22-25.

[28] Harris RD, Holtzman SR, Poppe AM. 2000. "Clinical outcome in female patients with pelvic pain and normal pelvic US findings." *Radiology*; 216(2):440.

[29] Barloon TJ, Brown BP, Abu-Yousef MM, Warnock N. 1994. "Predictive value of normal endovaginal sonography in excluding disease of the female genital organs and adnexa." *Journal of Ultrasound in Medicine*; 13(5):395.

[30] Sellors J, Mahony J, Goldsmith C, Rath D, Mander R, Hunter B, Taylor C, Groves D, Richardson H, Chernesky M. 1991. "The accuracy of clinical findings and laparoscopy in pelvic inflammatory disease." *American Journal of Obstetrics and Gynecology*; 164(1 Pt 1):113.

[31] Paavonen J, Aine R, Teisala K, Heinonen PK, Punnonen R. 1985. "Comparison of endometrial biopsy and peritoneal fluid cytologic testing with laparoscopy in the diagnosis of acute pelvic inflammatory disease." *American Journal of Obstetrics & Gynecology*, 1;151(5):645-50.

[32] Moore S. 2017. "Pelvic Inflammatory Disease." *Medscape*. URL: https://emedicine.medscape.com/article/256448-workup.

In: Pelvic Inflammatory Disease   ISBN: 978-1-53615-193-0
Editor: Daniel Abehsera   © 2019 Nova Science Publishers, Inc.

Chapter 6

PHARMACOLOGICAL TREATMENT

Azucena Molina[1],, MD, Isabel Lozano[1], MD
and Gemma Marín[1], MD*
[1]Obstetrics and Gynecology Department,
Quirónsalud Hospital, Málaga, Spain

1. INTRODUCTION

Pelvic inflammatory disease (PID) represents a spectrum of diseases with a wide range of severity. The challenge has always been to minimize sequelae of PID while not over diagnosing and hence over treating all women with genital tract symptoms with antimicrobials [1].

Treatment of PID must be empiric and provide broad coverage directed against the key pathogens. All regimens used to treat PID must be effective against *Neisseria gonorrhoeae and Chlamydia trachomatis*. Negative screening for these two organisms does not rule out upper reproductive tract involvement. Empiric coverage for anaerobic bacteria

---

* Corresponding Author's Email: azucena.molina@quironsalud.es.

should also be considered because they have been recovered from the upper reproductive tract in women with PID. Anaerobes, such as *Bacteroides fragilis*, have also been shown to cause epithelial and tubal destruction. The role of bacterial vaginosis in incident cases of PID is not clear. However, it has not yet been demonstrated that empiric antibiotics without anaerobic coverage leads to worse clinical outcomes [2].

Recommendations have been developed both in the United States and Europe for the management of PID with antibiotic therapy. These recommendations were based on the available evidence at the time, and the European guideline published in 2014 currently represent the most up to date evidence based guidance [3].

First and second-line inpatient treatments for PID differ between the guidelines. In the International Union against Sexually Transmitted Infections (IUSTI) guideline it is suggested that doxycycline should be given with oral metronidazole, whilst the United States Centers for Disease Control and Prevention (CDC) recommends this only if a tubo-ovarian abscess is present.

For outpatient regimens, there are differences in the recommended dosage of intramuscular ceftriaxone between the European and CDC guidelines. The higher dose of intramuscular ceftriaxone is recommended in the European guideline to reduce the risk of resistance developing in *Neisseria gonorrhoeae*.

Metronidazole is part of the recommended regimen in the European guideline, whilst for the CDC metronidazole is optional due to uncertainty of the importance of treating anaerobes. Oral ofloxacin or levofloxacin, plus oral metronidazole is a recommend outpatient antibiotic regimen in the European and CDC guidelines as long as the risk of gonococcal PID is low, reflecting the relatively high risk of quinolone resistance in gonorrhoea in many areas of the world. Oral moxifloxacin is not recommended in the CDC guideline but is suggested as an option in the European guideline if gonococcal PID is considered unlikely.

2. TREATMENT REGIMENS

Initiation of treatment is recommended as soon as the clinical diagnosis of PID is made. The most common criteria used to initiate empirical treatment for PID are the presence of pelvic or lower abdominal pain in a sexually active young woman in whom no other cause has been identified, and where one or more of the following criteria are present on examination: cervical motion tenderness; uterine tenderness; or adnexal tenderness. Additional criteria can be used to increase the specificity of a PID diagnosis (but decrease the sensitivity): oral temperature >38.3°C; presence of numerous white blood cells on saline microscopy of vaginal fluid; abnormal cervical or vaginal mucopurulent discharge; elevated erythrocyte sedimentation rate/C-reactive protein; and laboratory documentation of cervical infection with *Neisseria gonorrhoeae or Chlamydia trachomatis*. The absence of these additional findings does not exclude PID [3].

Admission for parenteral therapy, observation, further investigation and/or possible surgical intervention should be considered in the following situations: [4]

- Diagnostic uncertainty.
- Clinical failure with oral therapy.
- Severe symptoms or signs.
- Presence of a tuboovarian abscess.
- Inability to tolerate an oral regimen.
- Pregnancy.

In inpatients, the treatment response can be monitored by changes in C-reactive protein and white cell count. In severe cases and cases with failure of the initial treatment, tuboovarian abscess should be excluded by vaginal ultrasonography, computerized tomography or magnetic resonance imaging [4].

It is likely that delaying treatment increases the risk of long-term sequelae such as ectopic pregnancy, infertility and pelvic pain.

Because of this, and the lack of definitive diagnostic criteria, a low threshold for empiric treatment of PID is recommended (Evidence level IV, C) [5].

2.1. Recommendations for Inpatient Therapy

- Cefoxitin 2g/6 hours IV or cefotetan 2g/12 hours IV or ceftriaxone 1g/24 hours IV/IM plus doxycycline 100mg/12 hours IV [6] followed by oral doxycycline 100mg/12 hours and oral metronidazole 500 mg twice daily to complete 14 days (Evidence level Ia, A) [4].
- Clindamycin 900 mg / 8 hours IV plus gentamicin 240mg/24 hours IV [6] followed by either oral clindamycin 450 mg four times daily to complete 14 days or oral doxycycline 100mg twice daily plus oral metronidazole 500mg twice daily to complete 14 days (Evidence level Ia, A) [4].
- Intravenous therapy, should be continued until 24 hours after clinical improvement and then switched to oral [4].
- No difference in efficacy has been demonstrated between the recommended regimens [4].
- In our area, we prefer to use cafeteriaxone plus doxyclyne, plus metronidazole due to it being a more comfortable guideline, ceftriaxone is only administered daily.
- Alternative regimens: the evidence for alternative regimens is either less robust than the regimens above or they have a poorer safety profile based in the evidence.

  - Ofloxacin 400mg/12 hours IV plus metronidazole 500mg/8 hours IV for 14 days (Evidence level Ib, B).

- Ciprofloxacin 200mg/12 IV plus doxycycline 100mg/12 hours oral or IV plus metronidazole 500mg/8 hours IV for 14 days
  (Evidence level Ia, B) [4].

Oral administration of doxycycline is generally preferred, as soon as vomiting subsides, because of the pain associated with intravenous drug administration. Importantly, the bioavailability of the oral preparation of doxycycline is equivalent to parenteral administration [7].

Antiemetic and antipyretic medications should be offered to those patients who are symptomatic.

- Nausea or vomiting:

  - Metoclopramide 10mg/8h IV.
  - Rescue medication: Ondansetron 4mg/8h IV.

- Soft pain:

  - Paracetamol 1g/8h IV plus dexketoprofen 50mg/8h IV.
  - Rescue medication: Metamizole 2g/8h IV.

- Moderate pain:

  - Dexketoprofen 50mg/8h IV plus metamizoles 2g/8h IV.
  - Rescue medication: Tramadol 100mg/8h IV plus metoclopramide 10mg/8h.

Transitioning from parenteral to oral therapy can usually be started after 24 hours of sustained clinical improvement, such as resolution of fever, nausea, vomiting, and severe abdominal pain, if present [7].

Table 1. US and European current pelvic inflammatory disease inpatient treatment guidelines

	US Center of Disease Control and Prevention	International -Union against Sexually Transmitted Infections
Inpatient Regimen 1	Cefotetan 2 g IV /12 h (or cefoxitin 2g IV /6h) + Oral doxycycline 100mg/12 h for 14 days	Cefoxitin 2 gr IV/6 h (or Cefotetan 2 gr IV/12 h or Ceftriaxone 1 g IV or IM once daily) + Oral doxycycline 100mg/12 h /14 days + Oral metronidazole 500 mg/12 h for 14 days
Regimen 2	Clindamycin 900 mg IV/8h + Gentamicina IV/ 8 h (2 mg/kg of body weight) or 240mg IV/24 h + Oral doxycycline 100mg/12 h for 14 days or Oral dindamicine 450mg/6h for 14 days	Clindamycin 900 mg IV/8h + Gentamicina IV/ 8 h (2 mg/kg of body weight) or 240mg IV/24 h + Oral doxycycline 100mg/12 h for 14 days or Oral clindamicine 450mg/6h for 14 days + Oral metronidazole 500 mg/12h for 14 days
Regimen 3	Ampicillin/sulbactam 3 g IV/6h + Oral doxycycline 100 mg/12h for 14 days	Ofloxacin 400 mg IV/12h + Metronidazole 500 mg IV/8h for 14 days

2.2. Recommendations for Outpatient Therapy

- Ceftriaxone 500mg single dose IM followed by oral doxycycline 100mg/12 hours +/- metronidazole 400mg/6 hours for 14 days (Evidence level Ia, A) [4].
- Cefoxitin 2g IM single dose plus oral probenecid 1g single dose followed by oral doxycycline 100mg/12 hours +/- metronidazole 400mg/6 hours for 14 days (Evidence level Ia, A) [4].
- Alternative regimens:

  - Ofloxacin 400mg/12 hours oral plus metronidazole 500mg/12 hours oral for 14 days (Evidence level Ib, A) [4].
  - Levofloxacin 500mg/24 oral plus metronidazole 500mg/12 hours Ioral for 14 days (Evidence level Ib, A) [4].

Metronidazole is included in the recommended outpatients regimens to improve coverage for anaerobic bacteria, which may have a role in the pathogenesis of PID. Anaerobes are probably of relatively greater importance in patients with severe PID and some studies have shown good outcomes without the use metronidazole. In conclusion:

- Metronidazole should be added for patients with Trichomona vaginalis or in those women with a recent history of uterine instrumentation [7].
- Metronidazole should be discontinued in patients with mild or moderated PID who are unable to tolerate it [4].

Azithromycin has demonstrated short-term clinical effectiveness in one randomized trial when used as monotherapy (500mg IV single dose, followed by 250mg orally daily for 14 days), or in combination with metronidazole.

Table 2. US and European current pelvic inflammatory disease outpatient treatment guidelines

Outpatient Regimen 1	Ceftriaxone 250 mg IM in a single dose + Oral doxycycline 100 mg /12 h for 14 days +/- Oral metronidazole 500 mg/12h for 14 days	Ceftriaxone 500 mg IM single dose + Oral doxycycline 100 mg/12h for 14 days + Metronidazole 500 mg/12h for 14 days
Regimen2	Cefoxitin 2 g IM in a single dose + Probenecid 1 g orally administered concurrently in a single dose + Oral doxycycline 100 mg /12h for 14 days +/- Oral metronidazole 500 mg/12h for 14 days	Cefoxitin 2 g IM single dose + Oral probenecid 1 g + Oral doxycycline 100 mg/12h + Oral metronidazole 400 mg/12h for 14 days
Regimen 3	Oral levofloxacin 500 mg once daily or ofloxacin 400 mg/12h for 14 days +/- Oral Metronidazole 500 mg/12h for 14 days	Oral ofloxacin 400 mg/12h + Oral metronidazole 500 mg/12h for 14 days (ofloxacin may be replaced by levofloxacin 500 mg once daily)

In another study, it was effective when used 1g orally once a week for 2 weeks, in combination with ceftriaxone 250mg IM single dose. As of now, there is a lack of evidence in the use of azithromycin [3].

Women should demonstrate clinical improvement (e.g., defervescence; reduction in direct or rebound abdominal tenderness; and reduction in uterine, adnexal, and cervical motion tenderness) within 3 days after initiation of therapy.

If no clinical improvement has occurred within 72 hours after outpatient IM/oral therapy, hospitalization, assessment of the antimicrobial regimen, and additional diagnostics (including consideration of diagnostic laparoscopy for alternative diagnoses) are recommended [5].

3. PENICILLIN ALLERGY

The cross reactivity between penicillin and cephalosporin is < 2.5% in persons with a history of penicillin allergy. The risk for penicillin cross-reactivity is highest with first-generation cephalosporin, but is negligible between most second-generation (cefoxitin) and all third-generation (ceftriaxone) cephalosporin [5].

Treatment considerations must also take into account the risk for gonococcal infection [7].

3.1. Patients at Risk for Gonorrhea

Patients with PID who require hospitalization can be treated with clindamycin and gentamicin, as outlined above. However, therapeutic options for outpatient management of the penicillin allergic patient at risk for gonorrhea are limited, particularly among those with a history of severe penicillin allergy. In patients with mild or moderate PID, it is important to obtain a complete history regarding the underlying penicillin allergy so a therapeutic regimen may be constructed, as discussed below.

- History of mild allergy: patient with a mild past reaction to a penicillin and who never reacted to a cephalosporin (or never received one) may be a candidate for treatment with intramuscular ceftriaxone.
- History of severe allergy: Patients with severe or life-threatening penicillin allergies are not candidates for cephalosporin therapy, options for outpatient therapy are limited. It's recommended to administer a quinolone-based regimen (e.g., levofloxacin 500mg/24 hours orally for 14 days and a single dose of azithromycin of 2g orally), or hospitalize the patient and initiate endovenous treatment (previously mentioned).

3.2. Patients at Low Risk of Gonorrhea

As noted above, fluoroquinolones are not recommended for the treatment of PID because of the risk of gonococcal drug resistance.

However, fluoroquinolones, with metronidazole, may be considered for PID therapy in circumstances where *Neisseria gonorrhoeae* is not likely to be a causative agent (e.g., the post-menopausal woman who develops PID following uterine instrumentation). Thus, an alternate treatment regimen in these clinical scenarios may include levofloxacin (500mg/24 hours oral daily) or ofloxacin (400mg/12 hours oral daily) with or without metronidazole (500mg/12 hours oral daily), or monotherapy with moxifloxacin (400mg/24 hours oral daily), which has good anaerobic coverage, is another option. All regimens are given for 14 days.

Table 3. Gonorrhea risk factors

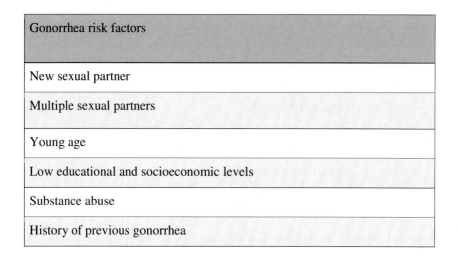

Gonorrhea risk factors
New sexual partner
Multiple sexual partners
Young age
Low educational and socioeconomic levels
Substance abuse
History of previous gonorrhea

4. Special Situations

4.1. Mycoplasma Genitalium

Mycoplasma genitalium is emerging as a cause of PID. In women, several studies have demonstrated the association between *Mycoplasma genitalium* and urethritis, cervicitis, endometritis, and pelvic inflammatory disease. In a recent meta-analysis, significant associations were found between *Mycoplasma genitalium* and cervicitis, and PID. *Mycoplasma genitalium* has been associated with preterm birth, and spontaneous abortion, but the prevalence in pregnant women in Europe is low, and therefore, the relative importance of this pathogen is probably small [8]. Azithromycin and moxifloxacin have in vitro activity against *Mycoplasma genitalium*, however, resistant cases are increasingly being detected.

Treatment of individuals with *Mycoplasma genitalium* urogenital infection prevents sexual transmission and is likely to reduce the risk of complications, including PID and tubal factor infertility.

Table 4. Treatment of Mycoplasma genitalium

Recommended treatment for uncomplicated Mycoplasma genitalium infection in the absense of macrolide resistance mediating mutations	· Azithromycin 500 mg on day one, then 250 mg /24 h 2-5 days. · Josamycin 500 mg/8 h for 10 days.
Recommended treatment for uncomplicated macrolideresistant Mycoplasta genitalium infection	· Moxifloxacin 400 mg/24 h for 7-10 days (oral).
Recommended second-line treatment for uncomplicated persistent Mycoplasma genitalium infection	· Moxifloxacin 400 mg/24h for 7-10 days (oral).
Recommended third-line treatment for persistent Mycoplasma genitalium infection after azithromycin and moxifloxacin	· Doxycycline 100 mg/12h for 14 days (poor efficacy, with microbiological cura rates between 30% and 40%) · Pristinamycin 1 g/6h for 10 days (oral)
Recommended treatment for complicated Mycoplasma genitalium infection (PID, epididymitis)	· Moxifloxacin 400 mg/24h for 14 days (oral).

Only few antimicrobial classes have activity against mycoplasmas including tetracycline, macrolides and fluoroquinolones [8].

4.2. Intrauterine Device

The use of intrauterine contraceptive devices (IUD) and risk for PID is primarily seen in the first 3 weeks after insertion and less so in those who are screened and treated for *Chlamydia trachomatis* and *Neisseria gonorrhoeae*.

According to CDC guidelines, the presence of an IUD should not alter the management of PID and there is no indication for immediate removal of the device.

However, if no clinical improvement is observed in 48–72h of appropriate therapy then there should be consideration for removal [2]. These studies primarily included women using copper or other non hormonal IUDs. No studies are available regarding treatment outcomes in women using levonorgestrel-releasing IUDs [5].

4.3. Pregnancy

PID in pregnancy, although uncommon, has been associated with an increase in maternal and fetal morbidity and preterm delivery. Management should be as an inpatient with parenteral antibiotics (e.g., ceftriaxone plus erythromycin plus metronidazole), although there is limited evidence to support any specific antibiotic regimen [3].

4.4. Pelvic Inflammatory Disease and Fertility

It is really important to aim an early diagnosis and treatment of PID before an irreversible damaged is caused to the Fallopian tubes. The risk of impaired fertility approximately doubles with each new presentation of PID and the use of condoms is advised to reduce the risk of recurrent infection [3].

4.5. Sexual Partners

Unprotected intercourse should be avoided until both partners have completed their course of antibiotics in order to avoid re-infection [3]. Partners should be advised to avoid unprotected intercourse until they and their partner have completed the treatment course.

The time interval for seeking partners is arbitrary, with the European guideline for the management of pelvic inflammatory disease recommending review of sexual partners within a 6-month period of onset of symptoms and the CDC suggesting assessment of partners within 60 days. The partners of patients diagnosed with PID should be referred for screening for gonorrhea and chlamydia and given appropriate empirical treatment (usually with azithromycin 1g single dose). If adequate screening for gonorrhea and chlamydia in the sexual partner(s) is not possible, empirical therapy for gonorrhea and chlamydia should be given [4].

4.6. Young Adults

No evidence is available to suggest that adolescents have improved outcomes from hospitalization for treatment of PID, and the clinical response to outpatient treatment is similar among younger and older women. The decision to hospitalize adolescents with acute PID should be based on the same criteria used for older women [5].

4.7. Menopause

In this age group the development of a tuba-ovarian abscesses seem to be associated frequently with serious pathology of the genital tract including coexisting malignant tumors, and the decision to treat a patient medically or even with conservative surgery may not be a safe option (up to 47% of the tuba-ovarian abscesses in menopausal woman should be a concomitant malignant cancer) [9].

4.8. Human Immunodeficiency Virus

Women with human immunodeficiency virus (HIV) may have more severe symptoms associated with PID but respond well to antibiotic therapy, although parenteral regimens may be required [5] so there is no difference between HIV-infected women with PID but the necessary of hospitalization [3].

5. PREVENTION AND COUNSELING

The mainstay in the prevention of PID is endorsing safe sex practices to decrease risk of transmission of sexually transmitted diseases. In addition, public health measures focusing on screening to control the transmission of *Chlamydia trachomatis* and *Neisseria gonorrhoeae* are essential. There is evidence that regular screening for *Chlamydia trachomatis* does reduce the risk of PID among young women.

Both the United States Preventive Services Task Force and CDC recommends screening for *Chlamydia trachomatis* and *Neisseria gonorrhoeae* in sexually active females aged 24 years or younger, and in older women who are at increased risk for infection (multiple or new partners or prior history of sexually transmitted diseases). The recommended screening intervals are not well defined [2].

Clinicians should counsel patients regarding the route of acquisition for sexually transmitted infections, the concomitant need for partner treatment, and future safe sex practices. All patients diagnosed with acute PID should be offered HIV testing. Other important components of the evaluation include:

- Assessment of immunity to Hepatitis B virus (e.g., through vaccination history or serologic testing) and vaccination of those who have no evidence of immunity.

- Serologic testing for syphilis.
- Patients who are 9 through 26 years of age should be offered immunization against human papillomavirus infection, if they have never been vaccinated in the past [7].

REFERENCES

[1] Llata, E., Bernsteing, K. T., Kerani, R. P., Pathela, P., Schwebke, J. R., Schumacher, C., Stenger, M., Weinstock, H. S. 2015. "Management of Pelvic Inflammatory Disease in Selected US Sexually Transmitted Disease Clinics: Sexually Transmited Disease Surveillance Network, January 2010-December 2011". *Sexually Transmited Diseases*, 42(8):429 - 433.

[2] Ford, G. W., Decker, C. F. 2016 "Pelvic Inflammatory desease". *Desease-a-Month*, 62:301 - 305.

[3] Duarte, R., Fuhrich, D., Ross, J. D. 2015. "A review of antibiotic therapy for pelvic inflammatory disease". *International Journal Antimicrobial Agents*, 46:272 - 277.

[4] Roos, J., Judlin, P., Jensen, J., International Union against sexually transmitted infections. 2014. "2012 European guidelines for the management of pelvic inflammatory disease". *International Journal of STD and AIDS*, 25(1):1 - 7.

[5] Workowski, K. A., Bolan, G. A., Centers for Disease Control and Prevention. 2015. "Sexually Transmitted diseases treatment guidelines, 2015". MMWR. Recommendations and reports: Morbidity and mortality weekly report. *Recommendations and reports/Centers for Disease Control*, 64:1 - 137.

[6] Polo, R., Palacios, R., Barberá, M. J. 2017. "*Documento de consenso sobre diagnóstico y tratamiento de las infecciones de transmisión sexual en adultos, niños y adolescentes*". [Consensus document on diagnosis and treatment of sexually transmitted

infections in adults, children and adolescents]. URL: https://www.seimc.org/contenidos/gruposdeestudio/geits/pcientifi ca/documentos/geits-dc-ITS-201703.pdf.

[7]   Up to date. 2017. "Pelvic Inflammatory disease: Treatment". Last Modified Jun. 2017. Accesed octubre 2017 https:// www.uptodate.com/contents/pelvic-inflammatory-disease-treatment/print.

[8]   Jensen, J. S., Cusini, M., Gomberg, M., Moi, H. 2016. "2016 European Guideline on Mycoplasma genitalium". *Journal of the European Academy of Dermatology and Venereology: JEADV,* 30:1650 - 1656.

[9]   Protopapas, A. G., Diakomanolis, E. S., Milingos, S. D., Rodolakis, A. J., Markaki, S. N., Vlachos, G. D., Papadopoulos, D. E., Michalas, S. P. 2004 "Tubo-ovarian abcesses in posmenopausal women: gynecologycal malinnancy until proven otherwise". *European Journal of Obstetrics and Gynecology and Reproductive Biology,* 114: 203 - 209.

In: Pelvic Inflammatory Disease   ISBN: 978-1-53615-193-0
Editor: Daniel Abehsera   © 2019 Nova Science Publishers, Inc.

Chapter 7

SURGICAL TREATMENT:
THE ROLE OF LAPAROSCOPY

Sadia Chocrón[1,], MD and Milagros Gálvez[1], MD*
[1]Obstetrics and Gynaecology Department,
Quirónsalud Hospital, Málaga, Spain

ABSTRACT

Nowadays, the treatment of the pelvic inflammatory disease (PID) has two purposes: short-term microbiologic and clinical cure (namely abdominopelvic pain, fever, leukorrhea and sickness); and long-term prevention of sequelae (namely tubal infertility, ectopic pregnancy and chronic pelvic pain) [1].

---

* Corresponding Author's Email: dr.s.chocron@gmail.com.

1. ANTIBIOTIC TREATMENT

Most of the cases of PID are resolved with antibiotic therapy alone, or antibiotic plus imaging-guided drainage procedures. 93% is the success rate of this conservative management [2]. Even the 95% of the tubo-ovarian abscesses are resolved with conservative management [3]. Only in a few cases surgery is necessary.

2. SURGERY INDICATIONS

2.1. First Intention (Immediate) Surgical Exploration

Surgical exploration on initial evaluation is indicated in the setting of an acute abdomen and signs of sepsis or hemodynamic instability, particularly if a ruptured tubo-ovarian abscess is suspected. Abscesses greater than 9cm can be considered candidates for immediate surgery, especially if they are complex or multi-cystic.

There is a direct relationship between the size of the abscess and the need for surgery, the poor evolution and the appearance of complications, as well as the increase in hospitalization time and the number of readmissions [4].

Postmenopausal women with tubo-ovarian abscess are at high risk of malignancy and surgery always should be considered.

If malignancy is confirmed complete surgical staging should be done.

2.2. Failure of Previous Treatment

Surgery is indicated if in 48-72 hours there is worsening or no improvement of fever, abdominopelvic pain, ileus, leukocytosis, size of abscess, as well if there are signs of abscess rupture or sepsis. It has been observed that women with endometriosis are more resistant to antibiotic treatment and often surgery is necessary [2].

2.3. Long-Term Sequelae Surgery Indications

Pelvic inflammatory disease can damage permanently the tubal tissues causing infertility and ectopic pregnancy. Chronic pelvic pain can be secondary to adhesion formation. Surgery has an important role in the treatment of these affections.

3. IMAGING-GUIDED DRAINAGE PROCEDURES

Imaging-guided aspiration and drainage is a feasible alternative to surgery in the treatment of pelvic collections. These procedures obviate general anesthesia, surgical wounds and associated surgical morbidity. Traditionally, interventional radiologists access the pelvic collections via transabdominal, transgluteal and endorectal approaches, guided by ultrasound, scanner or magnetic resonance.

The transabdominal approach usually entails long distances to the pelvic lesions and risks transgression of intervening viscera. The transgluteal approach risks damaging the nerves and vessels, and is occasionally obstructed by the pelvic bones. The endorectal approach is useful for accessing collections adjacent to the rectum but it is non-sterile [5].

Transvaginal approach was initially described in the early 1990s. The approach allows accurate, real time ultrasound-guided needle and drain placement, but has often been overlooked by interventional radiologists, owing to unfamiliarity and lack of data to guide case selection. Gynecologists are familiar with this approach. The Royal College of Obstetricians and Gynaecologists (RCOG) noted that ultrasound-guided aspiration of pelvic fluid collections may be equally effective as surgery, and this has been incorporated into the United Kingdom national guideline for the management of pelvic inflammatory disease since June 2011.

Studies have reported higher success rates for smaller, unilocular fluid collections. Thus, the multilocular nature of many complex tubo-ovarian abscesses collections may lessen the success rate in clinical practice [6].

We suggest the Seldinger technique for ultrasound-guided transvaginal drainage [7]:

- Prepare the patient with antibiotic therapy, analgesia and sedation.
- Empty the bladder prior to the procedure.
- Apply antiseptic solution in vagina and perineum.
- Place the transvaginal probe in the vaginal fornix and scrutinize the needle route for bowels, bladder and vessels. Upon confirmation of the needle route, advance the probe to stretch the vagina over the transducer head, and advance a 17 to 18 gauge needle into the collection under direct ultrasound guidance. If a drainge is indicated, insert a stiff 0.035 inch guidewire coaxially through the needle. Dilate the track and insert pigtail drainage catheter. Tape the drainage to the thigh and attach it to a urinary collection bag or a vacuum bottle. In an aspiration-only procedure, syringe the targeted fluid collection till emptied.
- Send all fluid specimens for microbiologic and cytological examination.
- Remove the catheter once the purulent output stops.
- Blockages of the drainage can be solved washing it with 5-10mL of saline solution -always with caution not to spread the infection to the entire abdominal cavity.

4. SURGICAL TECHNIQUE

4.1. Laparotomy Versus Laparoscopy

Regardless of the approach, the goal should be the same. The choice should be based on the expertise of the surgical team and the availability of the necessary equipment. Being a surgery that is expected to be highly complex - because of the extensive adhesions from the abscess to the surround structures and the necrotic and inflamed tissues surrounding the abscess - a large part of the gynecologists choose laparotomy because they have more ability to solve complications than using laparoscopy.

However, the laparoscopic approach seems to have improved outcomes of laparotomy, including decreased length of hospitalization, decreased rates of wound infections, and more rapid rate of fever defervesce.

4.2. Incisions

Low transverse incision like Pfannenstiel incision may be enough to expose the pelvis widely and solve abscesses located there. If an upper affection is suspected, a vertical midline incision can be extended easily to where it is needed.

If we consider the laparoscopic entry techniques overall, there is insufficient evidence to recommend one over another, and again the chose is surgeon dependent. An open-entry technique is associated with a reduction in failed entry when compared to a closed-entry technique, with no evidence of a difference in the incidence of visceral or vascular injury.

An advantage of direct trocar entry over Veress needle entry was noted for failed entry and vascular injury [8].

4.3. The Scope of Surgery and How to Proceed

Historically, most women with tubo-ovarian abscesses were managed aggressively with a total abdominal hysterectomy and bilateral salpingo-oophorectomy. Although this approach offered high cure rates, it was at the expense of high rates of surgical complications, infertility, and hormone deficiency. With the advent of effective antimicrobial therapy, operative management has become much more conservative moving towards procedures that allow for sparing of uterus and ovarian function.

We recommend the removal of the abscess cavity and the associated necrotic tissue - sending a sample for cultures - and then irrigation of the peritoneum. It is sensible to offer hysterectomy with bilateral salpingo-oophorectomy to patients who are acutely ill and have completed child bearing. This approach may hasten recovery compared with fertility-sparing surgery. In addition, this almost eliminates the need for repeat surgery.

Special mention for postmenopausal women in which the infection can be a consequence of cancer. In this context it is important to send tissue for histological study.

The mobilization of fixed and adhered masses can be very difficult. Scissor dissection is performed under direct vision. The surgeon should stay close to the tumor and away from the intestine. Adhesion traction facilitates dissection. The adhesions of the broad ligament and the pouch of Douglas can be released more easily with blunt dissection with the finger. It must be done carefully to avoid injuring the intestine, vessels or ureter, especially in dense adhesions where it is easier to injure them. When the mass has been released and the ureter has been identified, the infundibulopelvic ligament and mesosalpinx are clamped and dissected. Finally, the intramural portion of the fallopian tube is excised by wedge resection. In this surgery it is essential to identify the ureters, if there is any doubt it is better to dissect them because the most frequent complication is ureteral injury due to direct damage, contusion, and suture or adhesion formation [9].

4.4. Barrier Agents for Adhesion Prevention

Barrier agents have been suggested for adhesion prevention after gynaecological surgery.

There is no evidence on the effects of barrier agents used during pelvic surgery on either pain or fertility outcomes in women of reproductive age. Low quality evidence suggests that oxidised regenerated cellulose (Interceed), expanded polytetrafluoroethylene (Gore-Tex) and sodium hyaluronate with carboxymethylcellulose (Seprafilm) may all be more effective than no treatment in reducing the incidence of adhesion formation following pelvic surgery. There is no conclusive evidence on the relative effectiveness of these interventions. There is no evidence to suggest that fibrin sheet is more effective than no treatment.

No adverse events directly attributed to the adhesion agents have been reported [10].

Classically, after the extirpation of these adnexal masses, areas devoid of peritoneum must be covered with sigmoid colon, flap of peritoneum or omentum. Today it is a tendency to leave these areas open.

4.5. Drainages

Finally, we recommend placing a suction drainage in the cul-de-sac taking it out through the abdominal, and other supraaponeurotic suction drainage. They will be removed when there is clinical improvement and no purulent output.

REFERENCES

[1] Mitchell, C., Prabhu, M. 2013. "Pelvic Inflammatory Disease: Current concepts in pathogenesis, diagnosis and treatment". *Infectious Disease Clinics of North America,* 27(4):793 - 809.

[2] Habboub, A. Y. 2016. "Middlemore Hospital experience with tubo-ovarian abscesses: an observational retrospective study". *International Journal of Women´s Health,* 8:325 - 40.

[3] Lareau, S. M., Beigi, R. H. 2008. "Pelvic inflammatory disease and tubo-ovarian abscess". *Infectious Disease Clinics of North America,* 22(4):693 - 708.

[4] Dewitt, J., Reining, A., Allsworth, J. E., Peipert, J. F. 2010. "Tuboovarian abscesses: is size associated with duration of hospitalization & complications"? *Obstetrics and Gynecology International,* 2010:847041.

[5] Chong, L. Y., Toh, H. W., Ong, C. L. 2016. "Transvaginal Drainage of Pelvic Collections: a 5-year Retrospective Review in a Tertiary Gynaecology Centre". *Annals of the Academy of Medicine, Singapore,* 45(1):31 - 4.

[6] Beigi, R. H. 2017. "Management and complications of tubo-ovarian abscess". *Up to date.* URL: https://www.uptodate.com.

[7] Gu, G., Ren, J., Liu, S., Li, G., Yuan, Y., Chen, J., Han, G., Ren, H., Hong, Z., Yan, D., Wu, X., Li, N., Li, J. 2015. "Comparative evaluation of sump drainage by trocar puncture, percutaneous catheter drainage versus operative drainage in the treatment of Intra-abdominal abscesses: a retrospective controlled study". *BMC Surgery,* 9; 15:59.

[8] Ahmad, G., Gent, D., Henderson, D., O'Flynn, H., Phillips, K., Watson, A. 2015. "Laparoscopic entry techniques". *Cochrane Database of Systematic Reviews,* 31;8:CD006583.

[9]   Hirsch, H. A., Käser, O., Iklé, F. A. 2003. *Atlas de Cirugía Ginecológica* [*Atlas of Gynecological Surgery*], Madrid: Marban Libros.

[10] Ahmad, G., O'Flynn, H., Hindocha, A., Watson, A. 2015. "Barrier agents for adhesion prevention after gynaecological surgery". *Cochrane Database of Systematic Reviews,* 30;(4):CD000475.

In: Pelvic Inflammatory Disease   ISBN: 978-1-53615-193-0
Editor: Daniel Abehsera   © 2019 Nova Science Publishers, Inc.

Chapter 8

COMPLICATIONS AND CONSEQUENCES OF PELVIC INFLAMMATORY DISEASE

Marta García[1,], MD, and Celia Cuenca[1], MD, PhD*
[1]Obstetrics and Gynecology Department,
Quirónsalud Hospital, Málaga, Spain

1. INTRODUCTION

The clinical spectrum of pelvic inflammatory disease (PID) can lead endometritis, salpingitis, oophoritis, pelvic peritonitis, and perihepatitis and varies from the asymptomatic process to the vital commitment *(see clinical staging in chapter 2 "Clinical manifestations and diagnostic criteria").*

The major complications of PID are tubo - ovarian abscess (TOA), chronic pelvic pain, infertility, and ectopic pregnancy. Signs and symptoms associated with acute PID are poor predictors of the eventual

* Corresponding Author's Email: mgsanchez.mlg@quironsalud.es.

development of chronic sequels. Prompt diagnosis and treatment are important to reduce the risk of complications. However, even with timely treatment and clinical improvement in symptoms, or with a clinical or microbiologic cure of acute disease, long-term sequelae frequently occur.

Therefore clinicians should not assume that women with a complete recovery from PID have avoided the increased risk of long-term complications; this is thought to be secondary to the scarring and adhesion formation that accompany healing of infection-damaged tissues [1].

The risk of complications increases with the number of episodes and severity of PID. Options to reduce the risk of recurrence include the use of condoms and progestin-based contraceptives; however the protective role of oral contraceptives is controversial. Recurrent PID is associated with an almost two-fold increase in infertility and more than four-fold increase in chronic pelvic pain.

2. TUBO - OVARIAN ABSCESS

A TOA or pyosalpinx is a complex infectious mass of the adnexa that forms as a sequel of PID. Classically, a TOA manifests with an adnexal mass, fever, elevated white blood cell count, lower abdominal-pelvic pain, and/or vaginal discharge; however, presentations of this disease can be highly variable. In case of abscess rupture, potentially fatal sepsis can occur, so any clinical concern for this diagnosis requires prompt evaluation and treatment [2].

2.1. Epidemiology

Risk factors for a TOA are similar to those of PID and include reproductive age, intrauterine device insertion, multiple sexual partners, and a history of a prior episode of PID. The differential diagnosis for TOA often includes appendicitis, diverticulitis, inflammatory bowel disease, PID, ovarian torsion, ectopic pregnancy, ruptured ovarian cyst, pyelonephritis, and cystitis [2].

In 2002, the Center for Disease Control and Prevention (CDC) released new guidelines [3] for the evaluation and treatment of sexually transmitted diseases, which increased the number of patients being diagnosed with and treated for PID and reduced the prevalence of TOA from 20% to a mere 2.3%.

Human immunodeficiency virus positive women with PID generally have a slower clinical resolution of disease and therefore an increased risk for the development of a TOA.

2.2. Pathophysiology

Most commonly, these abscesses arise as a late complication of PID. Pathogens from the cervical infection or vaginal infection ascend first to the endometrium and then travel through the fallopian tubes into the peritoneal cavity where they form a walled-off mass. The majority of cases have associated peritonitis.

Bacteria from the lower genital tract ascend to create an inflammatory mass involving the fallopian tube, ovary, and potentially, other adjacent pelvic organs.

TOAs are often polymicrobial, and typically contain a predominance of anaerobic bacteria.

Although associated with sexually-transmitted infections, the most commonly recovered bacteria from a TOA include *Escherichia coli*, *Bacteroides fragilis*, other *Bacteroides* species, *Peptostreptococcus*, *Peptococcus*, and aerobic *Streptococci*. Interestingly, neither *Neisseria gonorrhoea* nor *Chlamydia trachomatis* is typically isolated from a TOA [2].

2.3. Evaluation and Management

A TOA can be found on imaging with ultrasound, computed tomography, or magnetic resonance imaging (Image 1 and 2). Laparoscopy is still considered the gold standard for diagnosing PID and TOA. Additionally, laparoscopy can facilitate the drainage and culture of a TOA. Due to its low-cost and lack of exposure to ionizing radiation, ultrasonography is an ideal imaging method to evaluate the concern for a TOA for women of reproductive age [2].

Typically, management consists of antimicrobial therapy *(see Chapter 6).*

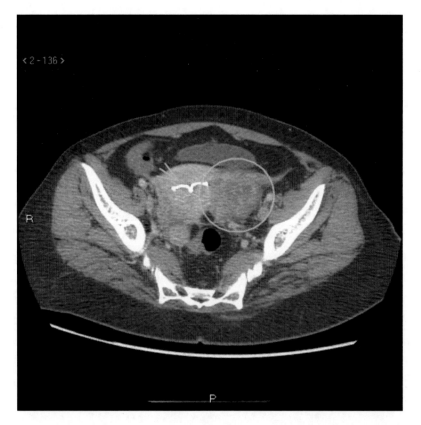

Image 1. Pelvis computed tomography with endovenous contrast. Heterogeneous left adnexal mass with inflammatory signs. Intrauterine device in endometrial cavity.

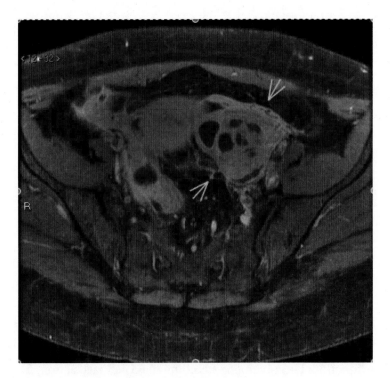

Image 2. Pelvic magnetic resonance, T1FS axial sequence with contrast.
Heterogeneous left adnexal solid-cystic mass that presents heterogeneous enhancement
and surrounding inflammatory signs compatible with tuboovarian abscess. The culture
was positive for Ureaplasma urealiticum sensitive to doxycycline. The intrauterine
device was removed and the evolution was positive after antibiotic treatment, resolving
the abscess.

Women with a TOA should be given parenteral antibiotics until
significant resolution, then antibiotics can be transitioned to an oral
regimen until there is complete resolution of the TOA upon repeat
imaging studies. Surgery is reserved for cases of suspected TOA rupture,
or cases with a poor response to antibiotics [2].

3. INFERTILITY: TUBAL INFERTILITY AND ENDOMETRITIS

The prevalence of infertility after PID is increased several-fold. This
rise depends upon multiple factors (chlamydial infection, delay in

seeking care for PID, recurrent PID episodes, severity of infection...).
Tubal factor is the main cause of infertility among woman desiring
pregnancy with a medical history of PID.

Subclinical PID, defined as histologic endometritis with no
symptoms of acute PID, appears to decrease subsequent fertility, even in
patients who are treated for chlamydia, gonorrhoea, and bacterial
vaginosis [1].

3.1. Tubal Infertility

The tubal factor is one of the main causes of female infertility
(approximately 30%) and indication of in vitro fertilization (IVF) cycles.
Both symptomatic and asymptomatic PID can cause permanent injury to
the fallopian tube, especially the endosalpinx (the mucosa of the fallopian
tube). There is a broad spectrum regarding the degree of severity of
anatomo-functional involvement including loss of ciliary action, fibrosis,
and occlusion. Hydrosalpinx represents one of the most severe clinical
forms and is defined as a distal tubal obstruction with lumen enlarged
and filled with sterile fluid (image 3, 4, 5).

The presence of hydrosalpinx exerts a clear negative effect on the
fertility of the patient and is also related to poor results in assisted
reproduction cycles [4].

Hydrosalpinx in patients undergoing IVF has negative consequences
on the rates of pregnancy, implantation, early pregnancy loss, preterm
birth, and live delivery. These findings described in IVF have also been
found in cryopreserved embryo transfers or in oocyte donation [5].

3.1.1. Why does Hydrosalpinx Reduce Fertility?

Strandell et al. believe that the hydrosalpinx fluid is of crucial
importance, but the actual mechanism of action needs to be
clarified [6].

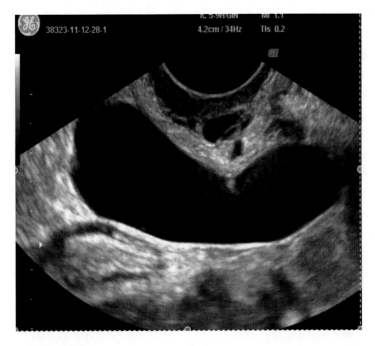

Image 3. Hydrosalpinx by ultrasound image.

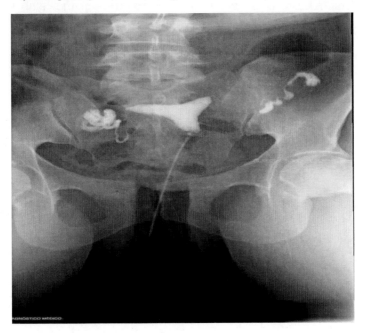

Image 4. Hydrosalpinx by histerosalpingography.

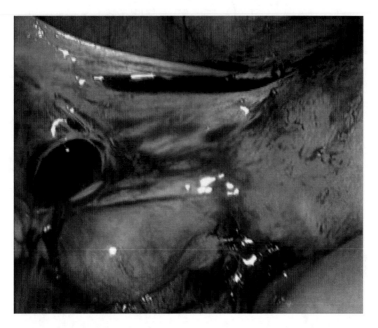

Image 5. Hydrosalpinx by laparoscopic image.

The main focus is on embryotoxic properties of the hydrosalpinx fluid, which include microorganisms, endotoxins, cytokines, oxidative stress and lack of nutrients.

The endometrial receptivity may be reduced as an effect of disturbed expression of the cytokine cascade, which is essential for implantation.

The presence of excessive fluid in the uterine cavity may also be a mechanical hindrance to implantation. The hydrorrhea has a clear negative effect, being able to produce a 'washed effect' of the embryo towards the vagina, diminishing the possibilities of apposition with the endometrium for the implantation.

In the other hand, the endometrial peristaltic activity, physiologically, increases in the first phase of the cycle and decreases in the luteal phase. Patients with hydrosalpinx show an increase in contractile activity of the uterus and this has been related to infertile cycles. These multiple mechanisms of action are produced in a parallel and not exclusive way.

3.1.2. In Vitro Fertilization Cycles

Outstanding advances in technology have made IVF an everyday treatment for infertility. The rapid development of IVF and embryo transfer has seen assisted reproduction proposed as a valid choice for women affected by different type of infertility including those with tubal factor. Assisted reproduction disregards the physiological role of salpinx during reproduction. But as we have already discussed in the previous paragraphs, it has been demonstrated that, in patients suffering from hydrosalpinx, the overall success of IVF is lower than expected. This led guidelines (e.g., NICE guideline [7]), and also supported by data analysed in a recent Cochrane review [8], to recommend laparoscopic salpingectomy (or at least tubal occlusion) before assisted reproductive technologies (ART) in case of signs or suspicions of hydrosalpinx.

While salpingectomy before ART is universally recommended in case of evident hydrosalpinx, no clear recommendations are available for the management of the wide spectrum of other tubal pathologies. The lack of accepted evidences regarding the potential detrimental effects of salpingectomy on ovarian reserve [6-10] further complicate the determination of the most appropriate management for tubal disease before ART. Available data suggested an absence of variation in ovarian reserve markers after unilateral salpingectomy while contradictory results were reported for bilateral surgery. Available data suggested an absence of variation in ovarian reserve markers after unilateral salpingectomy while contradictory results were reported for bilateral surgery.

Considering ART outcomes, data reported a significant improvement in on going pregnancy/live-birth rate in treated subjects without significant reduction in ovarian response to gonadotropin stimulation.

Further trials are needed to confirm the safety of bilateral salpingectomy on ovarian reserve, and to clarify the role of uni - or bilateral surgery in case of tubal blockage without hydrosalpinx.

3.2. Chronic Endometritis

Chronic endometritis (CE) is generally asymptomatic or has vague symptoms, such as abnormal uterine bleeding, pelvic pain, and leucorrhoea. Gynaecologists and pathologists often do not focus much clinical attention on CE due to the time-consuming microscopic examinations necessary to diagnose CE, its mild clinical manifestations, and the benign nature of the disease. However, the possible relationship of CE with infertility and/or perinatal complications has recently emerged as an area of on going research. In cases of CE the host immunity defends from microorganism, the distribution of lymphocytes involved in the implantation of embryos is altered, and ultimately, endometrial receptivity is reduced due to the inadequate secretion of various cytokines [11].

Endometrial interventions including hysteroscopic procedures *(Image 6)* and antibiotic treatment for CE could produce dramatic changes in future pregnancy outcomes [12].

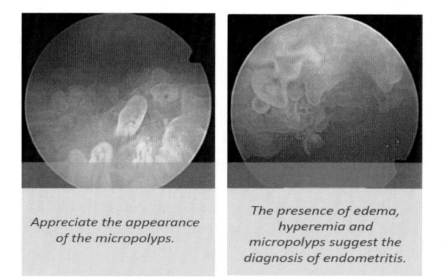

Appreciate the appearance of the micropolyps.

The presence of edema, hyperemia and micropolyps suggest the diagnosis of endometritis.

Image 6. Hysteroscopy diagnosis of cronical endometritis (Courtesy of Dr. Luis Alonso Pacheco. Hysteroscopy newsletter).

4. ECTOPIC PREGNANCY

Tubal damage caused by PID increases the risk of tubal pregnancy, as well as infertility. The increased expression of certain proteins involved in implantation may play a role in the pathophysiology [13].

Pelvic infection (e.g., nonspecific salpingitis, chlamydia, gonorrhoea), especially recurrent infection, is a major cause of tubal pathology and, therefore, increases the risk of ectopic pregnancy. Pelvic infection may alter tubal function and may also cause tubal obstruction and pelvic adhesive disease. Some data suggest that a history of chlamydial infection results in the production of a protein (PROKR2) that makes a pregnancy more likely to implant in the tubes [14].

The rising incidence of ectopic pregnancy is strongly associated with an increased incidence of PID.

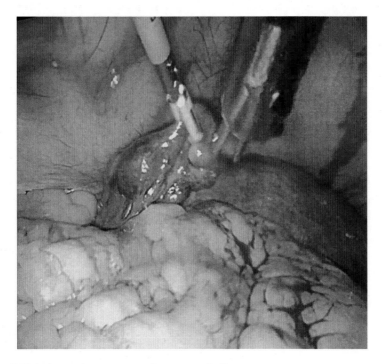

Image 7. Tubal ectopic pregnancy, Laparoscopic image.

Women with a history of PID have an approximately threefold increased risk of ectopic pregnancy [15]. In a prospective Swedish cohort study, the incidence of ectopic pregnancy in the first pregnancy after laparoscopically - confirmed PID was 7.8% versus 1.3% in women without PID at laparoscopy. The risk of ectopic pregnancy increased with the number of episodes and severity of PID [16].

5. CHRONIC PELVIC PAIN

Chronic pelvic pain (CPP) is defined as menstrual or non-menstrual pain of at least six months' duration that occurs below the umbilicus and is severe enough to cause functional disability. As many as 30% of women with PID develop chronic pelvic pain. While the precise etiology is unknown, the pain may result from scarring and adhesions that develop from inflammation related to the infectious process [1]. Therefore, PID is a common cause of CPP in settings with a high prevalence of sexually transmitted disease.

A study of risk factors for CPP in women with symptoms and signs of PID found recurrent PID was the strongest predictor for the development of this type of pain (odds ratio [OR] 2.84, 95% CI 1.07-7.54). Other risk factors included non-black race, married status, smoking, and poor mental health score [17].

A case-control study identified a correlation between a history of PID and painful bladder syndrome (OR 3.69, 95% CI 2.89-4.71), suggesting that painful bladder syndrome may be a squeal of PID [18].

Two factors correlate with the likelihood of developing CPP after an episode of acute PID: severity of adhesive disease and tubal damage (e.g., hydrosalpinx) and persistent pelvic tenderness 30 days after diagnosis and treatment [19]. However, the underlying reason that PID often leads to CPP has not been clearly established. In one study of 780 predominantly black urban women with recently diagnosed PID, those most likely to develop CPP were smokers, women with a history of two or more episodes of PID, and women with a low composite mental health score on standardized tests [20].

REFERENCES

[1] Peipert, J. F., Madden, T., Barbieri, R., Falk, S. 2016. *"Long-term complications of pelvic inflammatory disease"*. URL: https://www.uptodate.com.

[2] Kairys, N., Roepke, C. Abscess, Tubo-Ovarian. [Updated 2017 Oct 13]. In: StatPearls [Internet]. Treasure Island (FL): StatPearls Publishing; 2018 Jan-. URL: https://www.ncbi.nlm.nih.gov/books/NBK448125/.

[3] Centers for Disease Control and Prevention. 2015. "Guidelines for the treatment of pelvic inflammatory disease". In: *Sexually transmitted diseases treatment guidelines.* URL: https://www.cdc.gov/std/tg2015/default.htm.

[4] Camus, E., Poncelet, C., Goffinet, F., Wainer, B., Merlet, F., Nisand, I., Philippe, H. J. 1999. Pregnancy rates after in-vitro fertilization in cases of tubal infertility with and without hydrosalpinx: a meta-analysis of published comparative studies. *Human reproduction*, 14(5):1243 - 9.

[5] Tocino, A., Ferro Camargo, J. 2015. "Hidrosalpinx" [Hydrosalpinx]. In: García Velasco, J. A., *Cuadernos de medicina reproductiva, Cirugía Reproductiva;* 21(1):71 - 83.

[6] Strandell, A., Lindhard, A. 2002. "Why does hydrosalpinx reduce fertility? The importance of hydrosalpinx fluid". *Human reproduction*, 17(5):1141 - 5.

[7] National Collaborating Centre for Women's and Children's Health (UK). 2013. *"Fertility: Assessment and Treatment for People with Fertility Problems"*. London: Royal College of Obstetricians &

Gynaecologists. URL: https://www.nice.org.uk/guidance/cg156/ evidence/full-guideline-pdf-188539453.

[8]   Johnson, N., van Voorst, S., Sowter, M. C., Strandell, A., Mol, B. W. 2010. "Surgical treatment for tubal disease in women due to undergo in vitro fertilisation". *The Cochrane database of systematic reviews*, 20;(1):CD002125.

[9]   Noventa, M., Gizzo, S., Saccardi, C., Borgato, S., Vitagliano, A., Quaranta, M., Litta, P., Gangemi, M., Ambrosini, G., D'Antona, D., Palomba, S. 2016. "Salpingectomy before assisted reproductive technologies: a systematic literature review". *Journal of ovarian research*, 3; 9(1):74.

[10] Yoon, S. H., Lee, J. Y., Kim, S. N., Chung, H. W., Park, S. Y., Lee, C. 2016. "Does salpingectomy have a deleterious impact on ovarian response in in vitro fertilization cycles"? *Fertility and sterility*, 106(5):1083 - 1092.

[11] Cicinelli, E., Matteo, M., Tinelli, R., Lepera, A., Alfonso, R., Indraccolo, U., Marrocchella, S., Greco, P., Resta, L. 2015. "Prevalence of chronic endometritis in repeated unexplained implantation failure and the IVF success rate after antibiotic therapy". *Human reproduction*, 30(2):323 - 30.

[12] Park, H. J., Kim, Y. S., Yoon, T. K., Lee, W. S. 2016. "Chronic endometritis and infertility". *Clinical and experimental reproductive medicine*, 43(4):185 - 192.

[13] Quintar, A. A., Mukdsi, J. H., del Valle Bonaterra, M., Aoki, A., Maldonado, C. A., Pérez Alzaa, J. 2008. "Increased expression of uteroglobin associated with tubal inflammation and ectopic pregnancy". *Fertility and sterility*, 89:1613.

[14] Shaw, J. L., Wills, G. S., Lee, K. F., Horner, P. J., McClure, M. O., Abrahams, V. M., Wheelhouse, N., Jabbour, H. N., Critchley, H. O., Entrican, G., Horne, A. W. 2011. "Chlamydia trachomatis infection increases fallopian tube PROKR2 via TLR2 and NFκB activation resulting in a microenvironment predisposed to ectopic pregnancy". *The American journal of pathology*, 178:253.

[15] Weström, L., Joesoef, R., Reynolds, G., Hagdu, A., Thompson, S. E. 1992. "Pelvic inflammatory disease and fertility. A cohort study of 1,844 women with laparoscopically verified disease and 657 control women with normal laparoscopic results". *Sexually transmitted diseases*, 19(4):185 - 92.

[16] Li, C., Zhao, W. H., Zhu, Q., Cao, S. J., Ping, H., Xi, X., Qin, G. J., Yan, M. X., Zhang, D., Qiu, J., Zhang, J. 2015. "Risk factors for ectopic pregnancy: a multi-center case-control study". *BMC pregnancy and childbirth*, 15:187.

[17] Haggerty, C. L., Peipert, J. F., Weitzen, S., Hendrix, S. L., Holley, R. L., Nelson, D. B., Randall, H., Soper, D. E., Wiesenfeld, H. C., Ness, R. B. PID Evaluation and Clinical Health (PEACH) Study Investigators. 2005. "Predictors of chronic pelvic pain in an urban population of women with symptoms and signs of pelvic inflammatory disease". *Sexually transmitted diseases*, 32:293.

[18] Chung, S. D., Chang, C. H., Hung, P. H., Chung, C. J., Muo, C. H., Huang, C. Y. 2015. "Correlation Between Bladder Pain Syndrome/Interstitial Cystitis and Pelvic Inflammatory Disease". *Medicine*, 94:e1878.

[19] Trautmann, G. M., Kip, K. E., Richter, H. E., Soper, D. E., Peipert, J. F., Nelson, D. B., Trout, W., Schubeck, D., Bass, D. C., Ness, R. B. 2008. "Do short-term markers of treatment efficacy predict long-term sequelae of pelvic inflammatory disease"? *American journal of obstetrics and gynecology*, 198:30.e1.

[20] Haggerty, C. L., Peipert, J. F., Weitzen, S., Hendrix, S. L., Holley, R. L., Nelson, D. B., Randall, H., Soper, D. E., Wiesenfeld, H. C., Ness, R. B.; PID Evaluation and Clinical Health (PEACH) Study Investigators. 2005. "Predictors of chronic pelvic pain in an urban population of women with symptoms and signs of pelvic inflammatory disease". *Sexually transmitted diseases*, 32:293.

EDITOR'S CONTACT INFORMATION

Daniel Abehsera, MD, PhD
Coordinator of the Obstetrics and Gynecology Service
Hospital Quironsalud Málaga, Malaga, Spain
Email: danielabehsera@hotmail.com

INDEX

A

abuse, 40, 49, 50, 82
acid, xii, 31, 33, 38, 56
actinomycosis, 26, 46, 52
adhesions, ix, 4, 15, 62, 91, 93, 94, 95, 97, 100, 110
age, 5, 6, 7, 8, 27, 39, 40, 41, 42, 61, 82, 85, 87
anaerobic bacteria, 30, 53, 73, 79, 101
antibiotic, viii, 1, 8, 16, 20, 45, 57, 58, 60, 74, 84, 86, 87, 90, 91, 92, 103, 108, 112
antimicrobial resistance (AMR), xi, 33, 34, 35, 38
antimicrobial therapy, 94, 102
appendicitis, 22, 51, 63, 70, 101
assisted reproductive technologies (ART), xi, 107, 112
asymptomatic, 10, 12, 15, 27, 28, 29, 33, 34, 44, 99, 104, 108

B

bacteria, 19, 29, 44, 46, 47, 101

bacterial vaginosis, 7, 29, 46, 47, 48, 53, 68, 74, 104
bacterium, 26, 35
barriers, 44
bilateral, 3, 13, 14, 51, 63, 94, 107
bioavailability, 77
bleeding, 13, 18, 108
blood, viii, 20, 31, 44, 48, 57, 58, 60, 75,100
bronchopulmonary dysplasia, 29

C

cancer, 85, 94
candidates, 81, 90
Caribbean, 40
causal relationship, 8
center for disease control and prevention (CDC), xi, 5, 9, 19, 51, 74, 83, 85, 86, 101
cephalosporin, 80, 81
cervicitis, 12, 14, 28, 29, 31, 48, 57, 82
cervix, 8, 12, 14, 17, 32, 43
chlamydia, viii, 2, 8, 15, 19, 21, 25, 26, 27, 30, 31, 32, 33, 36, 37, 38, 40, 41, 43, 44,

46, 48, 54, 56, 58, 67, 73, 75, 83, 86, 101, 112

chlamydia trachomatis, viii, 2, 8, 15, 19, 21, 25, 26, 27, 30, 31, 33, 36, 37, 38, 43, 44, 46, 48, 54, 56, 58, 67, 73, 75, 83, 86, 101, 112

chronic endometritis (CE), xi, 67, 108, 112

chronic pelvic pain (CPP), ix, xi, 89, 91, 99, 100, 110, 113

clinical diagnosis, 18, 19, 55, 65, 75

clinical manifestations, v, vii, 11, 12, 13, 68, 99, 108

clinical presentation, 57

clinical staging, 16, 99

clinical syndrome, 33

complementary tests, v, viii, 55

complete blood count, 20, 57

complications, vi, 5, 12, 16, 27, 61, 70, 83, 90, 93, 94, 96, 99, 100, 108, 111

computed tomography, 102

computerized tomography (CT), viii, xi, 61, 62, 63, 64, 69, 70, 75

conjunctivitis, 28

consequences, vi, 35, 99, 104

contraceptives, xii, 40, 100

controversial, 44, 58, 100

correlation, 49, 58, 66, 110

cost, 2, 5, 9, 33, 35, 59, 102

counseling, 86

c-reactive protein (CRP), xi, 19, 20, 57, 61, 75

culture, viii, 21, 29, 30, 32, 33, 34, 35, 57, 61, 102, 103

cycles, 41, 43, 104, 106, 112

cyst, 59, 65, 101

cytokines, 106, 108

D

degradation, 47

demographic factors, 42

destruction, 4, 47, 74

detection, 9, 14, 17, 19, 30, 32, 33, 37, 57, 61

developed countries, 4

diagnostic criteria, v, vii, 11, 18, 19, 76, 99

differential diagnosis, 61, 63, 70, 101

discomfort, 12, 17, 55

diseases, 9, 10, 11, 15, 23, 36, 37, 38, 54, 56, 67, 68, 73, 87, 111, 113

disorder, 29

displacement, xii, 31

distribution, viii, 108

diverticulitis, 51, 101

drainage, ix, 61, 90, 91, 92, 95, 96, 102

drug resistance, 81

dyspareunia, 8, 13, 14

E

ectopic pregnancy, ix, 5, 22, 27, 28, 56, 76, 89, 91, 99, 101, 109, 110, 112, 113

ectropion, 43

emergency, 10, 61, 64

endometrial biopsy, 65, 66, 71

endometritis, xi, 2, 3, 11, 13, 23, 48, 53, 57, 59, 62, 66, 67, 68, 82, 99, 103, 104, 108

epidemiology, v, vii, 1, 4, 5, 10, 50, 53, 100

epithelial cells, 26

epithelium, 43

erythrocyte sedimentation rate (ESR), xi, 48, 57, 61, 75

etiology, viii, 26, 45, 56, 110

evidence, 15, 19, 22, 45, 57, 58, 64, 66, 74, 76, 80, 84, 85, 86, 93, 95, 112

evolution, 90, 103

examinations, 50, 108

exudate, 15, 17, 18, 20

F

fallopian tubes, ix, 2, 30, 39, 46, 47, 60, 62, 101
fertility, 84, 94, 95, 104, 111, 113
fertilization, xii, 104, 111, 112
fever, 14, 19, 29, 57, 77, 89, 90, 93, 100
first-generation cephalosporin, 80
fluid, 3, 4, 19, 31, 57, 59, 60, 62, 63, 64, 71, 75, 92, 104, 106, 111
fluoroquinolones, 57, 81, 83
formation, 2, 4, 15, 50, 51, 91, 95, 100

G

general anesthesia, 91
genitourinary tract, 28, 29
gonorrhea, 4, 8, 28, 41, 47, 48, 80, 82, 85
gram stain, 17, 35
growth, 26, 35, 43
guidance, 52, 74, 92, 112
guidelines, 23, 35, 67, 74, 78, 79, 83, 87, 101, 107, 111

H

hazards, 48
healing, 100
health, 28
health maintenance organization (HMO), xi, 49
high-risk women, 10, 31
history, 18, 34, 39, 44, 45, 49, 79, 80, 86, 101, 109, 110, 111
HIV, xi, 8, 46, 54, 56, 58, 61, 86
hormone, 94
hospitalization, 16, 20, 80, 85, 86, 90, 93, 96
human, 22, 28, 47, 69, 86, 87

human immunodeficiency virus (HIV), xi, 8, 22, 46, 54, 56, 58, 61, 69, 86, 101
hysterectomy, 94

I

image, 61, 62, 64, 65, 70, 104, 105, 106, 109
immune response, 44, 47
immunodeficiency, xi, 101
in vitro fertilization (IVF), xii, 104, 107, 112
incidence, viii, 10, 15, 29, 41, 44, 45, 48, 50, 93, 95, 109, 110
income, 42
individuals, 28, 49, 83
infection, xii, 2, 6, 8, 9, 12, 13, 16, 26, 27, 28, 30, 31, 33, 36, 39, 40, 43, 44, 45, 46, 47, 48, 50, 51, 52, 53, 54, 55, 56, 59, 61, 67, 68, 69, 75, 80, 83, 84, 86, 87, 92, 94, 100, 101, 103, 109, 112
infertility, 27, 28, 41, 43, 52, 76, 83, 89, 91, 94, 99, 100, 103, 104, 107, 108, 109, 111, 112
inflammation, 2, 3, 13, 15, 17, 18, 57, 62, 63, 65, 66, 110, 112
inflammatory bowel disease, 101
inflammatory disease, vii, xii, 1, 11, 22, 23, 25, 36, 39, 59, 68, 69, 70, 73, 91, 96, 113
initiation, 20, 53, 80
insertion, 15, 44, 45, 83, 100
international union against sexually transmitted infections (IUSTI), xii, 74
intervention, 27, 66
intra-abdominal abscess, 3
intramuscular (IM), xi, 35, 74, 76, 78, 80, 81
intrauterine divice (IUD), xii, 15, 17, 21, 40, 44, 45, 46, 58, 83
intravenous (IV), xii, 16, 58, 64, 66, 76, 77, 79

L

laboratory studies, 66
laboratory tests, 55, 56
Lactobacillus, 47
laparoscopic surgery, ix
laparoscopy, vi, ix, 15, 64, 65, 66, 70, 71,
    80, 89, 93, 102, 110
laparotomy, 93
leukocytosis, 19, 58, 90
lymphocytes, 108

M

magnetic resonance, 75, 91, 102, 103
magnetic resonance imaging, 64, 75, 102
management, vii, ix, 22, 34, 68, 74, 80, 83,
    85, 87, 90, 92, 94, 102, 107
mass, 4, 15, 16, 19, 61, 62, 65, 70, 94, 100,
    101, 102, 103
medical, 15, 36, 50, 52, 104
menstruation, 13, 40, 50
mental health, 110, 111
meta-analysis, 8, 82, 111
metrorrhagia, 13
microbiology, v, 25, 26, 36, 37, 68
microbiota, 46, 52
microorganisms, 2, 15, 47, 106
microscopy, 30, 56, 57, 75
models, 48
modifications, 44
molecular biology techniques, v, 25, 30, 35
monoclonal antibody, 32
mortality, 6, 9, 23, 37, 87
mucus, 18, 41, 44, 47, 50
multiple factors, 103
mycoplasma genitalium, 8, 9, 10, 25, 28, 35,
    38, 56, 58, 67, 68, 82, 83, 88

N

nausea, 77
negative consequences, 104
negative effects, 59
neisseria gonorrhoeae, viii, 2, 9, 15, 19, 25,
    28, 33, 37, 38, 44, 46, 48, 54, 56, 58, 68,
    73, 74, 75, 81, 83, 86
neutrophils, 3
nodules, 60
North America, 23, 38, 96
nucleic acid amplification test (NAAT), xii,
    30, 31, 32, 33, 34, 36, 38, 48, 56

O

obstruction, 4, 62, 63, 104, 109
occlusion, 104, 107
omentum, 95
oral contraceptives (OC), xii, 40, 43, 100
organ, 3, 7, 13, 18
organism, 31, 33, 34, 36, 46, 47, 67
outpatient, 4, 12, 16, 20, 21, 67, 74, 79, 80,
    81, 85
ovaries, 2, 39, 51, 60
oxidative stress, 106

P

pain, ix, xi, 1, 8, 12, 13, 14, 15, 17, 18, 19,
    23, 29, 48, 57, 60, 61, 63, 65, 70, 75, 76,
    77, 89, 90, 91, 95, 99, 100, 108, 110, 113
palpation, 14, 18, 19
parenchyma, 4
pathogenesis, 16, 30, 79, 96
pathogens, 25, 28, 42, 46, 47, 73
pathology, 9, 11, 61, 64, 70, 85, 109, 112
pathophysiology, 53, 109
pelvic inflammatory disease (PID), vii, viii,
    ix, xii, 1, 2, 4, 5, 6, 7, 8, 9, 11, 12, 13, 14,

15, 16, 17, 18, 19, 22, 23, 25, 27, 28, 29, 30, 36, 39, 40, 41, 42, 43, 44, 45, 46, 47, 48, 49, 50, 51, 52, 53, 55, 56, 57, 58, 59, 60, 61, 62, 63, 64, 65, 66, 67, 68, 69, 70, 71, 73, 74, 75, 76, 78, 79, 80, 81, 82, 83, 84, 85, 86, 87, 89, 90, 91, 92, 96, 99, 100, 101, 102, 103, 104, 109, 110, 111, 113

pelviperitonitis, 2, 4, 12

pelvis, viii, 3, 64, 93

penicillin, 23, 57, 80, 81

peptides, 47

perinatal, 108

perineum, 92

peripheral blood, 58

peritoneal cavity, 46, 101

peritoneum, 39, 62, 63, 94, 95

peritonitis, ix, 4, 11, 16, 22, 99, 101

pharmacological treatment, vi, 73

pharynx, 33

plasma cells, 3

pleurisy, 15

pneumonia, 15, 29, 35

polymerase, 31, 36, 37

polymerase chain reaction, 31, 36

population, 9, 29, 45, 49, 50, 53

pregnancy, 2, 15, 20, 56, 61, 84, 104, 107, 108, 109, 110, 113

pregnancy test., 56

preterm delivery, 84

prevalence, 4, 5, 6, 7, 8, 9, 10, 23, 29, 41, 43, 49, 51, 54, 82, 101, 103, 110, 112

prevention, xi, 5, 9, 19, 23, 36, 37, 41, 54, 67, 74, 86, 87, 89, 95, 97, 101, 111

probe, 32, 92

proliferation, 44

prophylaxis, 45, 52

protection, 43, 44

public health, 50, 53, 54, 86

pyelonephritis, 101

Q

quality of life, ix

R

racial differences, 40

radiation, 59, 61

reactivity, 47, 80

recommendations, 61, 74, 107

recovery, 94, 100

rectum, 33, 91

regenerated cellulose, 95

regimens, viii, 34, 73, 74, 75, 76, 78, 79, 81, 86

reproductive age, 6, 8, 95, 100, 102

resistance, xi, 33, 34, 35, 38, 57, 74

response, 47, 56, 58, 75, 85, 103, 107, 112

risk, vii, 7, 12, 16, 28, 33, 36, 39, 40, 42, 43, 44, 45, 46, 47, 48, 49, 51, 52, 53, 56, 57, 58, 74, 76, 80, 81, 82, 83, 84, 86, 90, 100, 101, 109, 110

risk factors, v, 7, 36, 39, 40, 42, 82, 110

S

salpingitis, 2, 3, 7, 11, 16, 37, 58, 60, 62, 66, 67, 69, 99, 109

salpingo-oophorectomy, 94

sensitivity, 13, 19, 30, 31, 32, 34, 36, 57, 59, 60, 66, 69, 75

sepsis, 13, 90, 100

serologic test, 86

sex, 27, 28, 33, 49, 86

sexual behavior, 40, 41, 42, 49

sexual intercourse, 6, 40, 42

sexually transmitted diseases, viii, 50, 58, 86, 101

sexually transmitted infection (STI), xii, 6, 7, 8, 12, 26, 28, 38, 39, 43, 45, 49, 51, 61, 86, 87, 88

signs, 15, 17, 18, 19, 20, 30, 57, 63, 68, 75, 90, 102, 103, 107, 110, 113

smoking, 7, 40, 49, 53, 110

Spain, 1, 11, 25, 39, 53, 55, 69, 70, 73, 89, 99

species (SPP), xii, 28, 35, 47, 101

sterile, 47, 91, 104

strand displacement amplification (SDA), xii, 31, 32

substances abuse, 40, 49

surgical intervention, 66, 75

surgical treatment, vi, ix, 58, 89, 112

susceptibility, 33, 44, 50

symptoms, vii, viii, 1, 11, 13, 14, 15, 28, 44, 46, 47, 57, 60, 61, 68, 73, 75, 85, 86, 99, 104, 108, 110, 113

syndrome, 15, 23, 63, 110

T

techniques, 30, 61, 93, 96

technologies, xi, 4, 107, 112

testing, 18, 27, 31, 32, 33, 34, 35, 37, 38, 50, 71, 87

therapy, 16, 20, 34, 46, 57, 58, 59, 74, 75, 76, 77, 80, 81, 84, 85, 86, 87, 90, 92, 112

thrombosis, 63

transcription - mediated amplification (TMA), xii, 31

transformation, 50

transmission, 28, 56, 83, 86

treatment, vii, viii, ix, 1, 2, 4, 8, 12, 16, 18, 20, 21, 22, 23, 26, 35, 36, 46, 49, 53, 54, 56, 57, 58, 60, 61, 67, 75, 76, 78, 79, 81, 84, 85, 86, 87, 88, 89, 91, 95, 96, 100, 101, 103, 107, 108, 110, 111, 112, 113

trial, 27, 36, 57, 67, 79

tuberculosis, 2, 26, 64

tubo – ovarian abscess (TOA), xii, 2, 4, 7, 99, 100, 101, 102, 103

U

ultrasound, viii, 19, 20, 59, 60, 61, 64, 69, 70, 91, 92, 102, 105

United Kingdom (UK), xii, 23, 34, 67, 92, 111

ureaplasma, 28, 29, 35, 37, 103

ureters, 94

urethra, 21, 32, 56

urethritis, 21, 30, 82

urinary tract, 14

urine, 31, 32, 33

uterus, 18, 29, 46, 51, 59, 94, 106

V

vagina, 2, 17, 92, 106

vaginal douching, 40, 48, 53

vaginitis, 29

vessels, 91, 92, 94

viscera, 51, 91

W

white blood cells, 57, 75

World Health Organization (WHO), 45

wound infection, 93

Y

young women, 26, 27, 50, 53, 86

Pelvic Pain: Causes, Symptoms and Treatments

Editor: Mary Montenegro

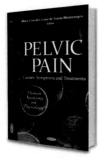

Series: Human Anatomy and Physiology

Book Description: In this book, the authors present topical research in the study of pelvic pain, including myofascial pain syndrome in the pelvic floor; hormonal modulation of genitourinary pain; the pathophysiology of endometriosis associated with pelvic pain; chronic non-bacterial prostatits; and physical therapy for women with pelvic pain.

Hardcover ISBN: 978-1-61324-656-6
Retail Price: $110

Alpha Lipoic Acid: New Perspectives and Clinical Use in Obstetrics and Gynecology

Author: Vittorio Unfer

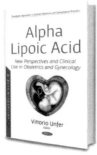

Series: Therapeutic Approaches in Common Obstetrics and Gynecological Disorders

Book Description: *Alpha Lipoic Acid: New Perspectives and Clinical Use in Obstetrics and Gynecology* focuses on the rationale of Alpha-Lipoic Acid (ALA) use in the field of maternal-fetal medicine and its clinical applications.

Hardcover ISBN: 978-1-53613-592-3
Retail Price: $160

PEDIATRIC AND ADOLESCENT SEXUALITY AND GYNECOLOGY:
PRINCIPLES FOR THE PRIMARY CARE CLINICIAN

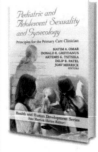

EDITORS: Hatim A Omar, Donald E. Greydanus, Artemis K. Tsitsika, Dilip R. Patel, and Joav Merrick

SERIES: Health and Human Development

BOOK DESCRIPTION: The book is written for practitioners by specialists, who are passionate about improving the future for our children and adolescents.

SOFTCOVER ISBN: 978-1-60876-735-9
RETAIL PRICE: $162